THE WOMAN WHO SWALLOWED HER CAT

THE WOMAN WHO SWALLOWED HER CAT

AND OTHER GRUESOME MEDICAL TALES

ROB MYERS, M.D.

Published by ECW Press
2120 Queen Street East, Suite 200, Toronto, Ontario, Canada M4E 1E2
416-694-3348 / info@ecwpress.com

LIBRARY AND ARCHIVES CANADA CATALOGUING IN PUBLICATION

Myers, Rob
The woman who swallowed her cat : and other gruesome medical
tales / Rob Myers.

ISBN 978-1-77041-061-9
ALSO ISSUED AS: 978-1-77090-077-6 (PDF); 978-1-77090-076-9 (EPUB)

1. Medicine—Miscellanea. 2. Medicine—Anecdotes. I. Title.

R706.M85 2011   610   C2011-902856-5

Editor: Randi Chapnik Myers
Cover design: David Gee
Text: Troy Cunningham
Printing: Webcom   1   2   3   4   5
ECW PRESS
ecwpress.com

The publication of *The Woman Who Swallowed Her Cat* has been generously supported
by the Canada Council for the Arts which last year invested $20.1 million in writing and
publishing throughout Canada, and by the Ontario Arts Council, an agency of the
Government of Ontario. We also acknowledge the financial support of the Government
of Canada through the Canada Book Fund for our publishing activities, and the
contribution of the Government of Ontario through the Ontario Book Publishing Tax
Credit. The marketing of this book was made possible with the support of the Ontario
Media Development Corporation.

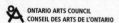

Canada Council   Conseil des Arts   Canadä   ONTARIO ARTS COUNCIL
for the Arts   du Canada   CONSEIL DES ARTS DE L'ONTARIO

PRINTED AND BOUND IN CANADA

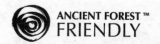

MIX
Paper from
responsible sources
FSC
www.fsc.org   FSC® C004071

ANCIENT FOREST ™
FRIENDLY

CONTENTS

INTRODUCTION

Some cases in forensic medicine are so bizarre, so unbelievable, bewildering and incomprehensible that they could not possibly be conceived in the imagination of a fiction writer or Hollywood producer. These cases are so disturbing that they have to be true. And the proof of their veracity lies in the sometimes dusty academic medical journal pages on which they are published. To find these fantastic stories, I spent countless hours scouring both recent publications and volumes that had gone untouched since they were first bound and shelved in medical library basements. Buried in thousands of obscure case reports spanning decades, an occasional case jumped out that was so strange, I found myself glued.

This book is a collection of fifty unbelievable and often disturbing cases of accidents, homicides, traumas, autoerotic fatalities, injuries and more. They are so mind-boggling that they seem made up. But although names have been changed, the medical facts have not. In fact, all of the following stories are culled from medical journals and based on real events — except for one.

Can you spot the one story in this book that is indeed a work of fiction? Go to ecwpress.com/myers to cast your vote.

DRAGON TALES

1

Sheldon learned his first card trick at age seven, and by fifteen, he considered himself an accomplished magician. Obsessed with learning more than simple sleight of hand, he spent his nights reading from books and practicing magic tricks on anyone and everyone. Like a drug addict, Sheldon needed progressively fancier tricks to fuel his passion. After a month of unsuccessful attempts to swallow swords, Sheldon turned to fire breathing in hopes of wowing his adolescent audience.

Small and socially awkward, Sheldon was an academic underachiever. As his math and science skills continued to disappoint his parents, he worked harder at magic, trying to gain approval, and even awe, from his peers. He hoped that breathing fire was a cool enough trick to boost him up the high school social ladder at least a couple of rungs.

Surprisingly, Sheldon picked up the art of fire breathing in no time. All he needed was to score some butane lighter fillers, mainly composed of isobutane. That was easy. He saved up his lunch money, and the next time his dad asked if he wanted to tag along to Home Hardware for windshield washer fluid and other household crap, he said sure. Then, in the store, he wandered around on his own.

How hard could it be, he thought, patting the lighters he had safely stowed in a bulge in his jean pocket under his sweatshirt. "A mouth full of lighter fluid, a lung full of air and I'm an instant dragon."

After a few weeks of practicing in his garage, singeing a few walls and burning some trash in the process, Sheldon was gaining popularity. After school, he was dazzling his new friends by swallowing small amounts of lighter fluid then morphing into a dragon before their very eyes. Flames leapt from his mouth in all directions.

"More fire breathing today?" Lester asked Sheldon as he passed him in the hall.

"Same place, same time," Sheldon said, referring to the alleyway a block east of Colton Junior High. He smiled, but his stomach hurt. Sheldon hadn't felt right for weeks. He was pale and nearly constantly dizzy. Even his parents noticed how sickly he had become. At first, he had treated himself with antacids with milk but in the last week or two, the concoction seemed to have lost its effectiveness.

When the bell sounded the end of the school day, Sheldon gathered his books from his locker. Standing with his combination lock in hand, he had to bend over as pain flashed through his belly, gnawing at him from the inside.

"You don't look so good," said Les, who was waiting to walk with Sheldon to the alley.

Lester, like Sheldon, was a bit player in the social games at school. But Lester's stable home life grounded him in confidence. The week he started ninth grade, Lester picked up on the stupidity of trying to look cool by abusing alcohol and drugs. A math whiz, he calculated that by staying straight and sober, his chances of addiction, teen fatherhood and early marriage would be far lower than that of his designer-clothes-wearing, beer-sneaking, unsupervised peers. And, of course, his dedication to karate helped him avoid the peer pressure that was closing in on some of his pals. The cool crowd knew better than to mess with Les. He confounded them with his quiet air of superiority, and of course, there was that darn black belt.

"It's this fire breathing stuff. I think it's dangerous," Lester told his friend. "Why bother with it? I mean it's all show. You and I both know the real skills are in your hands, and you're a great magician. You could get real paying gigs, man. Birthday parties, corporate events. Come on, buddy. It's time to put an end to this show-off stuff."

"That's what they told Houdini, Les," Sheldon replied, catching his breath. He stood up straight and managed a smile.

"See you soon, pal," Sheldon said, as he rushed to the bathroom down the hall. He locked himself into a stall, sat down, and exploded. He lay on his thighs, woozy again. After a few minutes, he stood up, pants around his ankles, and turned to look inside the bowl. There it was again. It looked like someone had dumped coffee grounds into the toilet. This had been going on for a couple of days now and guess what? He didn't drink coffee.

There was no time to stand around worrying. The show must go on, Sheldon thought, as he buckled up and high-tailed it down the hall and out the school doors to make it to his next performance. After all, he was the star.

Today, there was a small crowd bunched in the alley. Waiting, bored, a group of boys had amassed a mound of flammable trash in a Dumpster. When Sheldon ran up, they were kicking bottles against the brick wall.

"About fucking time, Superhero," said a tall boy with straight black hair shading his eyes. It was Tim, a popular kid from one grade up. "Keeping your fans waiting is a no-no."

Sheldon was an idiot, Tim thought. Then again, he thought everyone was an idiot. Destined to be either the CEO of a large corporation or a high-level cocaine dealer, Tim loved nothing more than directing younger kids into acts of violence. Lucky for him, Sheldon required little direction. Tim got a kick out of watching the skinny kid breathe fire like a dragon. His interest was, however, waning. He wondered what else he could cajole the sucker into doing.

Tim gripped Sheldon by the shoulder, a little too tightly. "Remember what we talked about, Shel. This'll be your biggest show of the season. See if you can cover the length of that pile of garbage over there and we can watch the entire alley go up in flames."

Sheldon was eager to please Tim, but the pain in his belly

was spreading like fire in a building doused with gasoline. Sweaty and light-headed, he glanced at Les. Then, turning his back to the crowd, he removed a small bottle of isobutane from his inside coat pocket.

After swigging an enormous mouthful from the pressurized container, Sheldon spun around, lifted his lighter and used his thumb to strike metal against flint. He turned to the crowd and spread his arms, making a great show of blowing the vaporizing liquid toward the flame. Aiming straight for the garbage, a huge river of fire erupted from his mouth and the crowd whooped and hollered.

Very few people noticed as the human flamethrower himself then collapsed on the concrete with a clunk.

Tim noticed, but didn't care. He was more interested in the crowd, standing mesmerized by the frenzied flames flying from the rusted Dumpster. Les raced to his friend's side. He pulled his cell phone from his pocket and, with shaky fingers, dialed 911.

Ten minutes later, the crowd heard the sirens and ran, leaving firefighters and paramedics to find a frightened Les and an unmoving Sheldon alone in the heated alley.

"I can't get a BP! Start a line!" a medic shouted. The team rushed in, inserting two intravenous lines that poured cold saline into Sheldon's veins.

"70 systolic. Let's move," the medic said. With that, the team bundled Sheldon into the back of the ambulance and sped to the hospital, leaving Les to explain the sequence of events to police.

Sheldon's blood pressure hovered dangerously low, while

his heart raced. Unstable, he was sedated, intubated and hooked up to a ventilator.

"He's bleeding," Dr. Dibin said in the emergency room. "Cross and type him and call gastroenterology, we need to get him scoped. Now."

Looking after kids made Dr. Dibin nervous. The boy was bleeding from somewhere inside, and based on the information the medics had relayed, it was obvious that the kid's esophagus, stomach and duodenum needed examining.

An hour later, Sheldon had lost half of his blood volume and desperately needed a transfusion. Through a subclavian line, the two units of fresh blood that hung above him in bags zipped through a tube and into his body.

Dr. Likornik, the on-call gastroenterologist, was equally fearful about caring for a teenager, but she had no choice. Sheldon couldn't be shipped to Sick Kids Hospital; he was too unstable. Steeling herself, the doctor arranged for an OGD to examine the boy's upper gastrointestinal tract.

As the patient lay sedated, Dr. Likornik inserted an Olympus high-definition flexible scope with a tiny camera on its end down his throat. Looking down the tube, she saw a flood of blood coating the mucosa of his esophagus.

Ingesting butane, a highly flammable component of natural gas, had caused Sheldon to suffer from a severe case of hemorrhagic esophagitis. It worked to freeze parts of his esophagus and stomach, killing the tissue and resulting in blood oozing from his esophagus and stomach, now home to a large bleeding ulcer. The ulcer was rhythmically ejecting blood into the stomach with every heartbeat. Via a port in the scope, Dr. Likornik used a needle to inject adrenaline into the source of bleeding. The drug constricted the blood vessel, damming the bleeding on impact.

It took two weeks before Sheldon had the strength to get out of bed. He had lost so much blood that his hemoglobin, which had dropped to 41, was among the lowest rates ever recorded in the hospital. The medical staff all agreed that while his recklessness had threatened to kill him, the boy's youth had saved his life.

In addition to heating, isobutane has some important functions, including refrigeration, and use as a propellant in aerosol cans. As for fire breathing, it's an activity that is surprisingly popular. It is described on the internet as a fun party trick that's not as dangerous as it looks and a surefire way to draw attention to yourself. But unless your goal is to gain the attention of coroners, fire breathing is best left to professional magicians, or, even better, to the dragons that made the term famous in the first place.

THE REMAINS OF THE DAY

2

Five years back, when her husband Chester first showed signs of dementia, Bea didn't think much of it. Eventually, though, it became clear that the man she had been married to for fifty-five years was a lot more absentminded than usual. The first signs were small: misplacing the keys to his tractor, wearing his nightshirt inside out, little mistakes like that. But Bea just attributed her husband's behavior to failing eyesight or the rusty mind that comes with age. After all, he was seventy-five years old. What did people expect?

But when Chester, a professional sheep farmer, forgot to graze the sheep, Bea knew there was something seriously wrong. He even forgot how to operate his Dixie Chopper zero-turn mower, and his acres of property quickly went wild when untended. Now that was unlike Chester, forgetful as he could be at times.

Perhaps more disturbing, Chester's naturally sweet disposition had turned surly and morose. He became incensed at the slightest perceived provocation. Usually up with the roosters, now Chester dropped into bed at dusk and slept past noon. Bea now knew, for certain, that this was not the Chester she had married and grown old with.

"We have to send in papers, Ma," said Becky, the oldest of Chester and Bea's four kids. "Otherwise he's gonna end up in hospital and we won't have choices. They'll send him wherever they darn well please."

"I know, honey," Bea replied. "But he was born and raised on this farm and this is his home. I can't just send him away, you know that. It would break my heart to see him in an institution."

And so, as is often the case with demented patients, Chester remained at home longer than he should have, barely recognizing his lifetime of possessions. And with her arthritis and metal hips constantly acting up, Bea was having a devil of a time keeping her eye on him.

Dementia refers to symptoms affecting cognitive function that result from the loss of brain cells. The condition is diagnosed when two or more central brain functions are affected. By then, the person has lost both intellectual and emotional ability; forgetfulness alone is not enough for a diagnosis. Today, more than ten percent of those over age sixty-five and half of people over eighty-five suffer from dementia.

The terms dementia and Alzheimer's disease are often used

interchangeably; however, Alzheimer's is but one cause of dementia. Other causes include Lewy body and Creutzfeldt-Jakob (mad-cow disease). The predecessors to these diseases — men with the names Alzheimer, Creutzfeldt, Jakob and Lewy — were all, oddly enough, German scientists. Another cause of dementia, indistinguishable from Alzheimer's, is multiple small strokes.

Sadly, as was the case with Chester, most forms of dementia are untreatable, eating away at personalities from the inside out. Very quickly — in just a matter of months — his personality seemed to fade to pale. Soon, the once vibrant, gentle farmer found himself reduced to a dependent 200-pound infant.

Chester, wearing a diaper, wandered around the farm. He started to pick up bits of food and garbage from around the property. It didn't matter what form the organic matter took; it was all food to him, and so into his mouth it went. By then, he had forgotten how to chew, though, so scraps just sat on his tongue, soaked in saliva.

Fearing Chester would choke and die, Bea lugged her robotic husband to the neurologist one last time.

"Mrs. Bleeker," Dr. Lavesky said, her chin propped on her hands. "I'm frankly surprised you're able to care for your husband at this point. His dementia is quite advanced. I think you have to seriously consider moving him to a home. There is nothing I can do here. There are no drugs to offer, no test. There is no cure."

Chester sat mute, his gaze empty. His brain was a tangled mass of confused neurons.

Bea sighed. None of this was news, but still, it was hard to hear.

"I am sorry to be so blunt," Dr. Lavesky said. "But you need to understand this situation. There is no hope for recovery. Dementia always gets worse. There are no drugs, no herbs and no diet that we know of to slow down the process in a meaningful way."

Bea's tears dripped onto her floral dress. Of course the doctor was right. Chester increasingly ceased to exist. The farm animals were more responsive to her than her own husband. In her heart, she knew that Chester had died long ago.

On the ride home, Chester sat in the passenger seat of his 1979 Dodge Dart, chewing his cheeks. In a flash of thought, Bea imagined driving straight off a bridge into the river. Now that would end their suffering. And yet, she wasn't sure that Chester was suffering at all. But she was. It was, she knew, time to do what she had always swore she would never consider.

A week later, Junior set to work lugging his father's belongings into Sunnyvale Retirement Home. There was Chester's worn wingback chair, the bureau he had built fifty years back, and a box of old, familiar clothes. In the lobby, Chester sat staring at urine-colored walls, a wad of pancakes still bulging in his cheek. Bea was at home, dusting. The thought of accompanying her husband to what would be his final resting place was too painful.

"Okay, Dad," Junior said with a grin. "You're all settled in. I'll come by soon." He knew he wasn't talking to the man he had known all his life. This was now just a shell of his wonderful father. Chester Junior thought he had accepted that fact years ago, but it still felt unbelievable.

It took a day for the staff at Sunnyvale to identify Chester's compulsive ingestion of just about any old thing, edible or not. Recently, Chester had graduated from organics to objects. In the absence of physical restraints, it was impossible to stop his compulsive behavior. The staff was constantly fishing stuff from his mouth: Kleenex (new and used), toilet paper (new and used), soap, and all manner of table scraps. Chester required twenty-four-hour observation, a luxury that Bea could not possibly afford.

Whenever nurses or orderlies heard choking, they rushed to find Chester, his throat clogged, his cheeks stuffed like an insatiable chipmunk.

Just two weeks after he arrived at Sunnydale, Chester awoke at 3 a.m. He was gasping for breath, but this time, the night nurse heard nothing. The following morning, another nurse chirped in with the sun, and stopped at the doorway. She almost vomited from the stink.

"Oh Lord," she said when she saw Chester. He lay cold on his single mattress, an island in a sea of feces. The smelly guck was all around his bed, and smeared on his mouth and nose. With excrement all over his face and hands, Chester looked like a child who had eaten chocolate pudding without a spoon, but that's not what he smelled like. Thankfully for the CPR staff, it was too late to breathe life into the patient's body via those lips.

Even the coroner's mask did a poor job of keeping the stench at bay. As is required for all unexpected deaths that occur in nursing homes, the coroner arranged an autopsy.

On examination, dissection of the upper airway identified the culprit: a 75-gram bolus of soft stool. The pathologist declined to analyze its origin, so regardless of whether it came from Chester's own diaper or the communal toilet, the cause of death on the postmortem examination read:

1. Upper airway obstruction from intentional ingestion of feces
2. Dementia
3. Obsessive compulsive disorder

Believe it or not, there is a medical term for the ingestion of feces: coprophagia. While autocoprophagics eat their own feces, allocoprophagics feast on the feces of others.

Since no one in his right mind would eat feces, the majority of patients who do so suffer from dementia or another form of organic brain disease or mental illness. More uncommonly, feces may be the food of choice for those with pica syndrome, which is characterized by unusual cravings for non-food items such as dirt (geophagia), glass (hyalophagia), mucus (mucophagia), wood (xylophagia), urine (urophagia) and metal items or food ingredients such as starch (amylophagia), salt or ice (pagophagia). The most unusual is geo-hyalomucoxylouroamylopagocoprophagia.

Chester died in a surprisingly undernourished state considering how often he shoved food into his mouth. The staff had done such a good job of removing objects from his grasp, it was a wonder he didn't eat himself. Although in the end, perhaps it can be said that he did.

STIFFED

3

With a snap of his latex gloves, Dr. Sheft signaled that he was done with the torso. He unrolled them from his hands and slipped on another pair, moving to the head of the table. After inspecting the brain, he would return the corpse to Refrigerator 6B.

Unfortunately, this autopsy failed to explain the cause of death. Here lay a twenty-year-old woman, dead in her prime, and the doctor saw no evidence of trauma — internal or external. Since she had suffered no obvious head injury, her brain looked normal, even though it had stopped sending signals via the spinal cord to her lifeless body. To determine whether or not there were drugs or other toxins in her system, the coroner would have to wait for the body fluid analysis results.

The pathology assistant, Ezra Montrose, or Monty as he

was known, set to work cleaning the corpse and stitching the large cuts in preparation for a postmortem examination.

Soon, the woman would be repatriated to her family, Dr. Sheft thought. She could be buried, cremated or tossed out to sea for all he cared. After decades of autopsies, he never considered what happened to corpses when his job was done. All that mattered to him was the cause of death. And that would be determined by body fluid analysis and the small snippets of organs to be placed in little plastic tubes of ten percent formalin for examination under the microscope.

She had been a beautiful woman, often described as Rubenesque, and she had been proud of her fashion sense. Her body had arrived decked out in $250 blue jeans paired with a designer top, and underneath, a lacy bra with matching thong. Now, her tattered, stained clothes were stuffed into a bright yellow collection bag tied at the top with a drawstring. It sat beside her pedicured toes (the color was called Yes I Can-Can, a jeweled shade of eggplant she had applied herself, humming, just the day before).

The woman's torso bore the typical upside down "Y" shaped incision, starting below her neck and traveling down the middle of her chest before branching diagonally along the inferior margin of each rib cage. Monty was busy stitching her organs into place with thick twine.

He had already sawed open her skull with a whirring blade. Bye-bye thousand dollar hair weave. Now Monty stopped his needlework to hand the woman's brain to the impatient doctor. Then he replaced the top of the skull as if he had just placed a candle inside a gutted jack-o'-lantern and his job was done.

With Mozart marching in the background, Dr. Sheft worked with the agility of an executive chef. Finding the gyri, sulci and fissures all in their proper places, he concluded that there was nothing amiss, but he went ahead and followed autopsy protocol, which required weighing every organ. He placed the brain on a Toledo vegetable scale.

Having finished his business, Monty awaited instruction from his master. He couldn't help but glance at the woman's naked corpse. Now that she was all sewn up, she actually looked pretty great, despite the damaged hair weave and absent brain.

Dr. Sheft's work done, it was time for Monty to hose down the body. This was his favorite part of the job, the final shower. This time, he sprayed longer than necessary before returning the woman to her temporary resting place in the corpse drawer of the morgue refrigerator. She would fit in the 1950 x 615 mm one designated for taller bodies. It was a stainless steel fabrication with an aluminum oxide interior and thermal insulating layer of polyurethane foam. It wasn't the Plaza, but hey, it still made for a reasonably comfortable bed, all things considered.

What had happened to this young woman? The doctor was stumped. Known in the morgue as JA16-2982010, she had been found in an alleyway behind a club rented out for massive rave parties held on the last Friday of every month. She was pulseless by the time the ambulance arrived. Dr. Sheft's presumptive diagnosis was simple: another drug overdose, likely Ecstasy, the flavor of the month.

Samples in one hand, his lunch in the other, the pathologist left the autopsy room and returned to his office. In the days it would take for the toxicology results to come back, he would conduct another four or five autopsies. People just never took a break from dying.

The following day, Dr. Sheft entered his office at precisely 8 a.m., as he had done every morning for the past twelve years. Within seconds, a technician appeared at his door, breathless.

"I think you need to come down to the cold room," she panted.

What now? Without a word, Dr. Sheft stood and strode through his office door and down two flights of stairs. At a large red door, he punched in his seven-digit security code on a keypad and swiped his index finger across the newly installed automated fingerprint verification system. Then he peered into the optical biometric scanner. Once he was recognized, a buzzer sounded, inviting him to enter. But when he stepped inside the brightly lit room, he froze. His assistant followed, stopping to stand right behind him.

Dr. Sheft considered himself a black-and-white man. In his world, there was simply no room for gray areas. You were either right or you were wrong, alive or dead. Because of this world view, and his robotic manner, the staff had nicknamed the doctor Data, after the sentient android on *Star Trek*. Although the nickname never made it to the doctor's face, it stuck. Word had gotten around.

"Bring the security tapes to my office, please," the doctor barked to his assistant. He was still facing the scene. His voice carried the authority that his diminutive stature could not.

Dr. Sheft knew enough to know this was an inside job. After

years sleuthing the cause of death through the examination of thousands of corpses, he was accustomed to detective work.

"I need an employee list that shows everyone in this hospital with access to the morgue," he said. "This is not something we can keep quiet. My secretary will contact the police. Please ensure that no one leaves the pathology lab pending their arrival."

Dr. Sheft drew in a deep breath through his nose and surveyed the scene. As ugly as it was, the fact remained that only a morgue professional would know that a crime had been committed overnight. To Dr. Sheft and the morgue assistant on duty, the horror before them was as clear as the open horizontal steel fridge and the naked body lying on the corpse drawer (or crisper, as it was affectionately known). A few rules had been broken:

Rule #1 — a body-laden crisper was never left open and unattended
Rule #2 — bodies, especially those belonging to voluptuous women, were never (ever) placed facedown on the narrow steel bed
Rule #3 — one body per crisper

Three hours later, Dr. Sheft was in the midst of a second autopsy on JA16-2982010, this time under the averted gaze of two young police detectives.

"There are signs of injury and tearing of the vulva," he stated, pointing to the woman's genitalia. "No blood."

He went on to explain: "Note that I performed an autopsy

on this body yesterday, and at that time, there were no genital lacerations. Note as well that lacerations bleed only in live people. These findings occurred post the postmortem, subsequent to yesterday's autopsy examination."

More senior police would have been immune to all manner of disgusting scenes. But the young detectives were already checking for washroom signs as they followed the doctor. With a cotton swab, Dr. Sheft collected a vaginal fluid specimen and carried the small glass tube to the microscopy room, located at the end of a long corridor. Rows of steel benches bordered a large rectangular table housing complex multi-headed microscopes. The doctor rubbed the swab on a clear slide and covered the specimen with thin glass, topping it like a sandwich. Then he slid the specimen under the scope. He twisted the knobs to bring the sample in focus.

"Okay, gentlemen. This is confirmation of the crime. All we need now is the perpetrator." And with that, he strode from the room, tailed by the nauseated detectives. They all ended up in Dr. Sheft's office. The young men could smell the rancid morgue odor clinging to their suits. Good thing they were $200 off the rack.

"Our system allows us to track all access to the holding area," the doctor explained. He held up a printout that the assistant had left on his desk. "As of my departure yesterday evening, only one subsequent entry was logged."

An hour later, police were dragging Monty into headquarters. They had surprised him at his apartment while he was frying eggs. A fully inflated realistic love doll sat on a kitchen chair watching the scene unfold. When told of the accusation against him, Monty shot his doll a loving look, rested his head in his cuffed hands and shook back and forth without a word.

In the small interrogation room, Monty sat facing one of the detectives.

"Listen, it wasn't me," he said.

The detective smiled like he was trying to pacify a young child. "Mr. Montrose," he said, enunciating the name. "The body was clearly violated and seminal analysis documented spermatozoa."

Monty looked blank, which exasperated the cop.

He raised his voice. "You know what that means, you sicko? Let me spell it out for you. Your sperm were found inside that dead woman. Now you didn't do her before she arrived at the morgue, did you?"

Monty wasn't about to dignify the question with an answer. Not without his lawyer, that was for damn sure.

"We have all of the evidence we need to lock you away for good," the detective said. Then he softened. "Now. If you want to man-up and confess, we may be able to work something out. This is a pretty huge burden, I bet."

Monty stared straight ahead. "Wasn't me," he said then he looked straight at the detectives. "You don't believe me? Go ahead. Test my DNA." He started to stand.

"Sit down!" yelled the detective, and Monty plopped back into the chair.

Within the hour, Monty was fingerprinted, issued a striped jumpsuit and led to a holding cell. He remained in the county jail, shaking his head and cursing, for a full week before the DNA results exonerated him as the necrophiliac.

Falsely accused and pissed off, Monty went straight from the courthouse to his lawyer's office. Burglary or vandalism was one thing, but being publicly accused of necrophilia by your boss, the most important pathologist in the state? Well, that bloody doctor was going to pay. This whole mess would cost the hospital a pretty pile of dough in severance and damages.

Dr. Sheft was perplexed, but not for long. He knew someone had screwed JA16-2982010. That much was obvious. He knew it wasn't him. And he knew that only one person had entered the morgue (and the corpse) after his departure. There was only one explanation. Monty had not been alone during his shift.

Fingering the DVDs on his desk, Dr. Sheft realized that he had the evidence right here. The entire scene had been caught on videotape via newly installed morgue surveillance. He had forgotten that the new system included this feature, and the young officers hadn't thought to ask about the presence of a videotape. He slipped the disc into the player, and there before him in color was Monty, entering the autopsy room, with a hooded man trailing close behind. Monty appeared to be giving a guided tour of the facilities.

Then, as Monty went to work sewing and hosing and preparing, his friend surreptitiously pulled out drawers and peeked inside before settling on JA16-2982010. All the while, Monty was occupied in a separate area of the morgue, oblivious to the man's activities.

Police knocked on the door of Monty's lawyer's office. They hauled Monty down to the station once again, where he watched the video, his fantasy of a future sipping piña coladas on a Mexican beach fading like the sunset. Why in hell had he let his cousin convince him to break protocol and bring him to work? Yes, his cousin was into vampires, but who knew that his fascination with the dead ran so deep?

Monty was fired yet again, this time with cause, while his cousin received a sentence of two years less a day with a mandatory psychiatric assessment.

Necrophilia is right up there with zoophilia (an "unhealthy" interest in animals) as the most grotesque of sexual perversions. Literally translated as "love of the dead," the term necrophilia was coined by a Belgian psychiatrist. Not surprisingly, most perpetrators are men who work in the death industry, in hospitals, funeral homes and cemeteries. Typically, the sex act occurs before burial, but not always, making for an even messier act for lovers of the dead.

BALL BREAKER

4

Matt was bored.

It was yet another night on the corduroy couch in front of the TV. This one just happened to be a Saturday. Leaning forward, he tore open another pack of Twinkies and shoved the sweet cake into his mouth followed by a plateful of spaghetti soaked in bottled tomato sauce, topped with parmesan cheese. He burped twice before collapsing back into the pillows. Matt loved food. So much so, that he wished he could eat lying down. Why was he always so bloody hungry? It was a mystery. One that wasn't worth tiring his brain out on.

He grabbed the TV remote and channel-surfed his way from the hockey game to the losers on *Intervention* to the local news. Like a kid with ADHD, Matt couldn't seem to focus. He clicked the remote every two seconds, feeding himself

Doritos straight from the bag. He washed the salt down with President's Choice iced tea. It was cheaper than the name brands and tasted a hell of a lot better than cold carbonated piss beer.

Matt hated the taste of beer. He preferred vodka to give him a head start on his Saturday evenings but he was all out. Tonight, he was off to hustle pool at the Sports Club. He was just having trouble getting his shit together.

For now, Matt let the remote slip to the floor and lay on his back, comatose on the couch. Car horns honked through the open window of his second-floor bachelor pad. The thin drapes, a remnant from the previous tenant, fluttered in the night breeze. He watched his distended abdomen move rhythmically up and down until his lids dropped. Hours passed. Matt snoozed. When he awoke, he tipped the bag of chips into his mouth like they were liquid. Then, as he had done every Saturday night at 10 p.m. for the past three years, he hauled himself off the couch, plucked his stained windbreaker from a chair, and zipped it over his Justice League T-shirt. Matt's entire wardrobe was made up of vintage T-shirts including pictures of cereal boxes, *Star Trek* themes, *Sesame Street* characters and of course, his beloved superheroes.

On his way out, he checked his teeth for food in the hallway mirror and shut the apartment door behind him. Too lazy to walk down two flights, he waited ten minutes for the rickety elevator to find his floor. On the street, he jumped into a cab. He was heading into another late night refuge from his hazy, bloated and unemployed existence.

Just six minutes later, Matt was inside the Sports Club.

Without traffic to fight, it would have taken him the same amount of time to walk. But exercise just wasn't his thing.

The bar was a mix of picnic tables covered in checkered cloths. There was an impressive collection of chewed gum stuck to their undersides. On top, pitchers of draft beer and plates loaded with heart-threatening nachos and wings fought with condiments for space. Booths ringed the perimeter of the room. Hanging from the corners, flat-screens shone with a variety of televised sports games. At the back stood four Winchester pool tables. Solid maple with majestic carved legs, each retailed for 24 grand.

The only women in the room were young waitresses dressed in tight V-necks and matching short shorts, outfits their mothers would be horrified to see them wearing — let alone in a bar full of drunk, rowdy men.

As he strode toward the pool tables, Matt nodded to familiar faces: Paul, Mark, Prabhat. Like Matt, his friends were unemployed, overweight and clad in faded superhero T-shirts in shades of gray, brown and bile green. They all wore sweatpants with adjustable drawstrings and dirty sneakers that were older than the waitresses.

Despite his hatred of beer, Matt ordered a Molson Dry, tilted it back and sucked the bottle clean. He called for two more then elbowed through the crowd, thrilled by the sound of the pool balls clacking off each other. Ah, the comforts of home.

Then he spotted his friend. "Yo, yo, yo! Bookmeister!" he called.

Dave Bookmeister sat with his back against the wall. He

was so large that it was hard to see the chair beneath him. He was hunched over, his stubby fingers wrapped around a pool cue. "Hey," Dave said, his face vacant.

"So where's the action tonight?" Matt whispered into Dave's ear. He was looking for what is known in pool circles as a mark.

Matt had very few life skills. He didn't cook, he didn't clean, he didn't exercise, work, or drive. But he had one skill that those who didn't know him would never have guessed. Matt was a serious pool shark. Hustling and unemployment insurance paid Matt's rent and kept him living large. And for that, he was grateful.

To answer his friend's question, Bookmeister nodded in the direction of a clean-shaven man in his late twenties one table over. Matt squinted at the stylized tattoo on the side of the man's neck, and watched him rest his cigarette on the edge of the table, a definite no-no. The man then lined up his shot before missing what to Matt looked like an easy corner. The man straightened up, glanced over and scowled at Matt.

"What the hell are you looking at?" he called.

Matt gave him a loopy grin and shrugged, hoping to draw the unsuspecting asshole into a game. After all, this place was his territory. And tonight, he planned to fill his pockets with some serious coin.

Over the next hour, Matt's mark proceeded to lose game after game. The stakes were small, though. Too small. Pretty soon, Matt was sure. This asshole was not unsuspecting after all. He knew a lot more about pool than he was letting on. It was all there: in his too awkward pose as he held the cue, the way his eyes twinkled when he missed, the smooth strokes that were obviously too wide. Yes, Matt decided, it was very clear. This mark was hunting for a mark of his own.

Players drifted in and out, until it was Matt's turn. He dropped his coins into the slots and waited for the balls to flow. Matt racked them up, purposefully fumbling as he arranged them inside the triangle.

"So what are we playing for?" he asked.

"Your call," the mark said.

Both marks coolly anticipated fleecing the other. They decided on ten bucks, a safe, calm start. But soon, with both players trying to hide their skills, frustration mounted. Balls ricocheted off each other and missed pockets. After fifteen minutes and no clear leader, Matt's opponent stopped.

"Okay, pal, let's cut the bullshit," he said, offering a challenge: "You think you can beat me? Four hundred bucks says you can't."

Staring at Matt, he slapped the bills on the table and folded his arms across his chest.

Hmm, four hundred was a lot of Twinkies and spaghetti, Matt thought, feeling his belly gurgle. This bet was triple his usual stakes. Matt was ready. Sure, he didn't know how good the guy was. But hey, when Matt's high school buddies had been studying algebra, he was at the pool hall, doing his own kind of homework.

The problem was that Matt didn't exactly have four hundred bucks in his pocket. He had only half. So he spent a few minutes cajoling his friends out of the rest. And the bet was on.

A crowd gathered to see who would win the snooker game with the high stakes. The marks flipped a coin and Matt broke.

Five minutes was all it took. Matt, elated, went to scoop up the bills.

"Not so fast," the mark said, grabbing Matt's wrist. "Best two out of three."

"No way," Matt countered. "Deal's a deal." He could already taste those Twinkies. Matt was confident. This was his turf. The mark's eyes roamed the room. Recognizing no one, he stepped back.

"How about another bet?" the mark asked. "A hundred says I can stick a cue ball in my mouth and drink a beer around it."

"What kind of stupid bet is that?" asked Prabhat who had come to stand alongside his friend with a half dozen others. "Why would anyone pay you a hundred bucks to prove you're a moron?"

"Tell you what," Matt said. "I'll give you a chance to win fifty bucks back. It sounds like such a ridiculous stunt, that for entertainment alone, it's worth the bet." He slapped the bill on the table. "But you buy your own beer."

The mark came back with a Budweiser. He quickly stuffed the white ball in his mouth and proceeded to down the entire bottle. If Matt hadn't seen it with his own half-drunk eyes, he wouldn't have believed it. He was still up 350 bucks, and man, fifty bucks was a bargain for that show. But how the hell did the guy do it? It looked mighty easy, that's for sure.

Matt was starting to feel the effects of the beer. He was giddy, at ease, a showman. "Now it's my turn," he said for the benefit of the crowd.

He picked a red ball off the table and shoved it into his mouth. Far. Too far. He tried to pinch it, grab it back, but it was slipping down his throat. Made of smoothed phenolic resin, the ball was too big, too round and too smooth.

With the back of his throat completely occluded, Matt was silent. He couldn't even gag. Panicked, he reached toward the crowd with both hands, like a zombie, until he started falling toward his friend Paul. Paul turned Matt around and wrapped his arms around his generous girth, in a desperate attempt at the Heimlich maneuver. But the ball wouldn't budge.

Matt's eyes grew wide as the ball. Staring straight ahead, his last image was of a smirking, tattooed mark.

Someone called 911 and the paramedics struggled through the crowd. Using a laryngoscope, they tried to create an airway with an endotracheal tube, but were met with a cue ball around which not even air could pass. It didn't matter, though. Matt's body was already stiff.

That night, instead of lying on his cozy couch, Matt lay naked on a stainless steel autopsy table. Using a special surgical instrument, the pathologist worked for just a few moments before dislocating Matt's jaw and extricating his killer. The final report concluded that the death was caused by asphyxiation with a pool ball — also known as death by misadventure.

THE DISAPPEARING MAN

5

"*I Got You Babe . . .*" *Sonny and Cher sang straight into Wade's* dream. Eyes shut, he reached over and slammed the snooze button on his clock radio. Then he pulled himself up to a sitting position, scratched his balls through his underwear and yawned. Time to go. He stood and made his way to the bathroom. The dawn had barely broken through black night. A truck driver, Wade was accustomed to early mornings and long days awake.

After his shower, Wade brushed his teeth, rubbed on deodorant and tiptoed in his towel to the bedroom closet. Once there, he closed the door to keep the light from waking his wife, and donned his work shirt and trousers. Across his right breast pocket sat the company name: ALKALIES CHEM-ICAL.

Before heading downstairs, Wade mouthed "I love you" to the closed doors of his kids' bedrooms. In the kitchen, he poured a glass of milk and peeled a banana. Then he disarmed the alarm pad, nearly tripping on a school bag on his way out the door.

Inside his truck, Wade chugged through the humid morning. The cylindrical chlorine tank the truck carried looked like a white opaque water bottle for an office cooler, only thousands of times larger. It was tied by a series of ten thick iron chains, each of which Wade had ensured was tightly secured the night before. The tank was filled with 2,500 gallons of concentrated sodium hypochlorite solution, otherwise known as pool chlorine.

With one hand steadying the oversized wheel, Wade lit a cigarette. The cab was his second home, only much quieter without the kids around. And better, sometimes. Early in their marriage, his wife had banned smoking from the house, so this first morning drag was nothing short of ecstasy. Wade had tried to quit a dozen times, using nicotine patches, medications, even hypnosis. But he was still addicted. Although he felt guilty that he couldn't shake the filthy habit, the monotony of driving for hours on end in an enclosed space sure didn't help the cause.

Thirty minutes into Wade's journey north, the brakes hissed and the truck rested at a quiet intersection. When the light turned green, he shifted gears. But as the rig lumbered on, a horn blared, shocking Wade alert. A Chevy Impala flew across his path, swerving in a near miss, just inches in front of the truck. Wade pulled his siren and cursed the jerk who had nearly cost him time and money, neither of which he had enough of as it was. Swerving around the Impala, he flipped the driver his middle finger.

As his heart began to slow, Wade carried on, only to spot the car in his rearview mirror. It was accelerating. "Oh, give me a break," he said aloud as if the driver could hear and would listen to reason.

The roads were still quiet and the sun was on the rise. The car shadowed the truck, honking and swinging in erratic S-shaped paths. Wade drove slowly and methodically, hoping the guy would get his thrills and just give up.

"What the hell?" Wade called in vain. "I'm driving thousands of pounds of lethal cargo and you want to fight?"

Behind him, the frenzied driver shifted into the lane of oncoming traffic to position himself beside the cab of Wade's truck. Honking and gesturing, the madman seemed like he might slam his car into the truck's side, a fight Wade would surely win. Then, almost out of nowhere, another car appeared, driving toward them from the opposite direction.

To avoid a head-on collision, the approaching vehicle had no choice but to veer into the ditch beside the road. Now Wade was genuinely scared. He was safe inside the rig. But if he stopped, despite the size of his truck, he may be in danger. Reports of road rage came through the radio all the time. There was no way of knowing if this maniac had a baseball bat on the seat beside him, or worse, a gun.

The guy had already demonstrated that he had no respect for human life. Pitying anyone who happened to be on the road, Wade knew what he had to do. He would drive straight to the police station with the madman in tow.

Abandoning his route, Wade turned the truck to the right, and the car followed. But to his chagrin, he found himself on a road under construction, narrowed to a single lane through which traffic took turns traversing over about fifty yards. He slowed to a halt. Then, glancing out the window, he saw a hand shoot up, grab his side mirror, and there, staring into his eyes, was the face of a lunatic. His adversary, all bloodshot eyes and scruffy beard, banged like an animal on the window, nearly cracking the glass.

"Get the fuck out!" yelled the nut. "Get the fuck out!"

Wade panicked. He fixed his eyes forward, deftly shifted gears and jammed the accelerator hard. Luckily, he was at the front of the line. The rig lurched forward and the psychopath's feet flew out from under him. He held onto the mirror with both hands.

Picking up speed, Wade focused on just one word: escape. After three full minutes with his feet flying off a mirror on a straightaway, the man registered no fear. Instead, he started spitting on the window.

Wade needed him off his truck, and fast. He spun to the left. The outside wheels leapt off the ground as the other tires squealed. The man tumbled back, landing with a splat on the road just before the chlorine tank shook ten iron chains and shifted over, carried by centrifugal force. Free from its restraints, the tank rolled onto the man's chest, trapping his flailing limbs under a load of sodium hypochlorite. His yells came out muffled as he squirmed and tried to escape becoming roadkill.

The pool chlorine inside the tank was composed of a mixture of chlorine and a fourteen percent solution of sodium hydroxide. It was powerful, with a pH of 13.5, which, even when diluted in water, could irritate the skin if it was not properly dissolved before contact.

Lying trapped beneath the tank, the man might have lived. Assuming a car didn't smash into the tank before the police arrived, it could have been rolled away by a team of men. Likely, the crazy man would have suffered broken ribs, perhaps a concussion from the fall. To recover, he would need a couple of weeks in hospital, and maybe even a stint in rehab.

It wouldn't have been so bad, and not likely fatal, had the seam in the tank not ruptured, leaking rivers of burning chemical over the man, showering his limbs, and eroding skin, muscle and tissue in a matter of seconds. As he screamed, the chlorine corroded his femurs, tibias and fibulas and ate into his marrow, bleaching his bones white as Wade watched, horrified, from the safety of his cab.

Snapping to, Wade jumped down to help, but the fumes rose and spread, overpowering the air, forcing him away from the tank. So he stood just ten feet back, witnessing the man who had wanted him dead melt faster than the Wicked Witch of the West.

Emergency personnel arrived. But without chemical suits, they could not get near the tank either. Fire crews pulled out their hoses, and tried spraying the chemical with water. But even as they were trying to save the man, they watched the tissues of his lower torso disappear.

Twenty minutes later, a Level 5 crew, replete with impermeable self-contained hazard suits, arrived on the scene. Together, the men removed the tank, and dragged away what was left of the disappearing man.

The pathologist, who was near retirement, thought he had seen it all. But with the reek of chlorine eclipsing the usual odors of formaldehyde in the basement pathology department, it was the first autopsy he had to perform with a gas mask.

The report showed that the man's legs and pelvis were free of all soft tissue and muscles. His white bones looked like they had been exposed to decades of desert heat. His genitalia were nearly gone. A skull fracture was noted, likely sustained when he fell on the road from the height of the rig's cab.

Following autopsy routine, the lab analyzed both blood and body fluid. Not surprisingly, Wade learned, the man had been acting under the influence of high levels of alcohol and cocaine. Aha.

THE SANTA SYNDROME

6

Keith's Sporting Emporium occupied the northeast corner of a concrete strip mall in a small Arizona town. It was a nondescript cinderblock of flaked white paint, housing an assortment of sports goods ranging from lawn darts to shotguns.

From the day Keith's took up residence on the outskirts of town where the rent was low, it was a target. Protected by window bars, a reinforced steel door, motion sensors and light beams, the store was an impenetrable fortress to the addicts and hooligans who loitered outside it after midnight.

Spencer had been planning his caper for weeks. He intended to lower himself into the store after hours and load as much prized merchandise as he could into the back of his truck parked out front. It would all come down on the Easter long weekend when the store would be closed.

Finally, the Saturday of the big heist came. At 3 a.m., when night was at its blackest, Spencer leaned a ladder against the back wall of Keith's. He climbed up, crept toward the chimney, and removed the metal grate intended to deter birds. He peered into the sooty hole.

Spencer had cased the store half a dozen times. To keep the manager from getting suspicious, he always bought some cheap item — a plastic duck decoy, fishing lures, a street hockey stick. In the meantime, he knew exactly what to steal. When the big day came, he would fill his backpack with as many hunting knives as he could fit, and with a couple of golf bags full of brand new clubs slung over his shoulder, he would burst out the front door and make his getaway. Spencer knew a guy in Phoenix who was interested in the merchandise. He would drive straight there, and have cash in hand before the next morning.

First though, fancying himself an expert thief, Spencer took his time exploring the doors and windows, and noted the location and type of alarm he would have to deal with. The system was complex and with sensors on all entry points, he knew that without the code, he was a dead duck the moment he opened a door or window.

Oh glory day when Spencer discovered that the motion sensors were absent from the back room, which was impossible to access without walking through the store. Unless, of course, you slid down the chimney.

At age thirty-four, Spencer was an unskilled career crook. He had been arrested eight times and had spent two years in the tank for burglary. Just one more conviction and he'd be rotting for years in the state penitentiary. This heist, though, was different. No one would expect a robbery through the chimney. That was Santa Claus's turf. Well, Christmas was here early this year.

Spencer checked his simple gear — a coiled rope knotted here and there in several places to allow for easy ascent and descent, a backpack, some rusted tools. The night air was hot and still. The light of the half-moon spilled Spencer's shadow across the building's flat roof. He tied the rope around the chimney and threw the end down the hole. It fell to the floor with a plop. Sweating, grunting and as usual, just a little bit drunk, he lowered himself into the grate.

A daily beer guzzler since the age of seventeen, Spencer was no longer lithe. In fact, his now doughy waist seemed to grow about two inches per year. And yet, Spencer didn't seem to notice. When he looked in the mirror, he still saw the skinny kid he was teased for being in eighth grade.

Squeezing down the chimney, Spencer was eager for his feet to find the floor. But before he knew it, his right hand was stuck, wedged between his ear and the chimney brick.

"Fuck!" he whispered, feeling beads of sweat pop in his armpits.

I can do this, he thought, wiggling his legs, trying to drag down his arm. But now his ankle was stuck, too. What the hell was he going to do?

Luckily, it was early Sunday morning, so no one would turn a key in the door lock for more than twenty-four hours. But by 6 a.m., the numbness in Spencer's arms and legs turned to searing pain. Pretzeled, his limbs began to swell, cementing him inside the chimney, and mounting pressure in his muscles and tissues.

As the high from the beer wore off, Spencer became scared. Suddenly, his fear of being discovered transformed into a fear of not being discovered. Like an animal caught in a cage, he began to whimper.

"Help! Help!" he called as light shot down from above, soaking him in sweat. It was getting hard to breathe as stale soot filled his lungs.

Throughout the day, the townsfolk sang hymns in church and enjoyed their ham dinners at home, while a mummified Spencer lapsed in and out of consciousness. Over and over, he soiled his pants, but the stench had no effect on him in the haze of his brick prison. By late Sunday, he had no more urine left.

The first thing Keith noticed, even before he stabbed the code on the elaborate alarm he had installed just last year, was the smell. After the holiday Monday, the store had been closed for two and a half days.

Perhaps some clever squirrel had found his way in and then died somehow, he thought, but then the alarm would have sounded and the company would have called him at home. Maybe it was mice. Or garbage left to rot.

Keith rushed around the store, grabbing an N-95 mask off the Aisle 12 shelf along the way and strapping it on against the stink. In the back room, there it was. A wet mess of urine and poop in a disgusting pile on the chimney floor. A coyote must have somehow found its mark from the roof of the building, he thought, cursing at the fact that his week would start with scrubbing clean all traces of the excrement with bleach. Well, there goes the weekend, he thought, as a rustle sounded from above. Was the animal stuck in the chimney? Maybe he should light a fire and roast the sucker. That would teach him.

Instead, Keith dialed the local pest removal service. A half hour later, a late model Chevy van swerved into the parking lot. On its side was an emblazoned photo of a raccoon under the motto *No Job Too Big or Small.*

"There are raccoons in Arizona?" Keith asked the driver.

"Not anymore," the guy said, showing his teeth. Outside the store, Keith told the man about the smell, the excrement, the sound, and his conclusion.

The man was confused. "What the hell would a coyote be doing on your roof?" he asked.

The two circled the building. At the back, a battered old Ford F-150 stared at them. Spencer had forgotten to move his getaway truck to the front parking lot. Near the truck, leading up to the roof, sat the ladder.

"I better call the cops," Keith said.

Soon, fire and ambulance personnel were at the scene, and a policeman was perched on the ladder's top step. He shouted down into the hole.

"Hey, you!" he called. Barely conscious, the echo reverberating in his head like ripples of water, Spencer reached for the sound. He mumbled as his eyes rolled back.

Fortunately, Spencer had not made it far, so after smashing the upper bricks with a sledgehammer, the rescue team hooked his swollen body and hauled it up and out.

A medevac helicopter transferred Spencer to the regional

trauma center. En route, his breathing began to slow and a long plastic tube, inserted into his lungs to open his airway, helped. But by the time he arrived on the helipad, his blood pressure had plummeted. Intravenous lines pumped liter after liter of crystalloid fluid into his body.

In the intensive care unit, Spencer lay on a stretcher. The main muscle groups of his body were now gangrenous and infected. His limbs were swollen to three times their normal size causing further pressure within his damaged tissues, a condition known as compartment syndrome.

Five days later, the doctors had no choice but to amputate Spencer's arms and legs. Overwhelmed and poisoned by the myoglobin released from his dead muscles, his kidneys failed. Just one week after he was saved, Spencer suffered a cardiac arrest and died.

Spencer fell victim to the little known Santa Claus Syndrome where a person becomes accidentally trapped in a chimney, air duct or heating vent, and suffers, as a result, positional asphyxia, compartment syndrome, and often, burn injuries. Within eight hours of being trapped, muscle death begins. Almost all cases involve ill-fated attempts at burglary. So here's a message to all you would-be Santa Clauses out there: if you want to steal, do it the old-fashioned way — by smashing a window or jimmying a door. You're more likely to survive, even if you do end up rotting in jail.

ITALIAN STALLION

7

One sticky morning, when he was thirteen years old, Chad awoke from a wet dream and from that day on, he was hooked on masturbating. He considered himself the sole (or palm) player in a one-man orchestra; a virtuoso on the skin flute; a concert penis. If he had studied languages with as much dedication as he applied to playing with himself, Chad figured he would be fluent in both Spanish and Japanese by now.

Like most teens, Chad enjoyed video games, skateboards and a good frequent whack. He furtively hid his adolescent habit under the covers late at night and again, early in the morning. His closest companions included boxes of supersoft tissues, socks and the downstairs toilet. He had never been caught with his pants down by anyone. Thank God.

By age nineteen, Chad had grown from a bored adolescent

into a bored young man. He was a high school grad, living at home, holding down a part-time job at Business Depot. One night, he called his buddy Len.

"What's up?" he asked. "Wanna head down to Screeches and hang?"

"Naw," Len said. "I'm stayin' in. Gotta get up early tomorrow for work. I was out late last night with Jenny and I'm still hungover."

"Come on, wuss," Chad chided. "Hell, it's Friday night."

"No can do, Bud. It's late. Go watch porn." Len laughed and hung up, leaving Chad holding the phone, frustrated.

In Chad's world, boredom easily slipped into the urge to masturbate. It was his Pavlovian reflex.

At 10 p.m., his parents out at yet another dinner party, there Chad sat, alone on the faded leather easy chair in the basement. He slouched into it, facing the TV. This chair, stained with tomato sauce and body fluids, was his own personal work of art. Only he knew how those stains got there. Hand down his pants, he channel-surfed through crappy late-night shows for an hour before heading upstairs for food.

Chad opened and shut kitchen cabinets, hunting for jars of Prego. It was time for his late-night pasta special. He twisted off the lid, dumped the tomato sauce into a bowl and shoved it in the microwave. After a few minutes, he loaded a handful of uncooked spaghettini into a pot of boiling water. The thinner the pasta, the sooner it was ready.

Chad liked his pasta cooked limp. Al dente? What was that? He strained the mass in a colander then forked it into the steaming bowl of sauce. He dumped a load of Parmesan cheese onto his creation. Standing, shoveling clumps of food into his mouth, a bizarre idea came to him. He grabbed a fistful of uncooked rods of pasta. He thought they might come in handy.

"Nothin on," he muttered from the comfort of his leather chair. "Should've rented a flick."

With one hand feeding his mouth noodles, and the other playing with his noodle, it was inevitable. Overloaded with pleasure, Chad began to develop an erection. Blood raced to the cylindrical chambers of his penis, and Chad continued to rub. But as erect as he was, he could tell somehow that he was not even close to coming.

Figuring this might just do the trick, he grabbed a raw rod of spaghettini and examined it. It was so erect, so smooth. He ran his fingers up and down its skinny shaft, feeling it, caressing it. Finally, in one bold move, he inserted the stick into the slit of his penis.

Immediately, Chad bolted upright and yelped in pain. He grabbed the stick to remove it but as he did, it broke, with one end lodged inside his now limp penis. The burning sensation began to build, until Chad thought he might be on fire inside. Tears spilled down his cheeks. He jumped up and started hopping around like a rabbit.

"No! No! No!!!" he screamed. He knew full well that there would be no way to extract the spaghetti on his own. He had to pee. But just the thought of urinating nearly made him faint.

Pain shooting through his midsection, Chad rushed around for the phone. He dialed emergency services. Waiting for the operator, he worried about what he would say. Clearly, he could not explain his situation. Shame flooded him and he hung up, sobbing now in fits and sniffles on the floor.

Within minutes, though, he realized he had no choice. He had to go to the hospital. Now.

Keys in hand, Chad ran to the car and eased himself inside. Somehow, he found the will to press the accelerator and steer the wheel. Somehow, he found himself pulling into a parking space in the hospital lot.

Limping into the triage area, he approached the glass.

"Appendix," he squeaked to the nurse, as he doubled over in pain. Seeing Chad's distress, she hurried to get him to a waiting bed.

The intern whisked into the room. She consulted her notes then smiled at Chad with even teeth. "So you're experiencing abdominal pain on the left side?" she asked. With four years of medical school behind her, she was still new to the field. Despite his agony, Chad could not help but notice her breasts straining against her buttoned blouse. His mind unbuttoned her shirt and released her twins. He winced.

"Uh, that's not really the thing," he whispered. "Actually my cock is killing me. The burning is too much."

"Excuse me?" the intern asked, confused.

Chad coughed. She was smoking hot. He tried not to stare but he couldn't help it. The pain was constant and severe. A nine on a pain scale of ten. He was going to have to tell the truth. Confess. Spill.

"Um, I just said it was something else because of what happened," he said, dancing around the problem. "I was messing around I guess, and it got out of control."

The intern nodded. She had no idea where he was going with this story. But in four years, she had seen a lot of blood, a lot of gore. How bad could it be?

He's kind of cute, she thought. Young but definitely cute.

"I, uh, I put something inside my cock I shouldn't have," he said. "And it's killing me!"

The intern blushed. Apparently, she still had lots to see in this job. "Well, let me get my staff," she said, trying to sound casual before scurrying from the room.

"Great," thought Chad, lying back on the bed, trying to distract himself from the pain. Her staff is going to examine my staff.

Within minutes, a bearded doctor appeared. Wearing hospital greens and a stethoscope around his neck, he introduced himself as Dr. Tyberg.

Chad was simultaneously relieved and disappointed that the doctor was a man.

"Dr. Prentice here says you may have inadvertently introduced a foreign object into the introitus of your member?" the doctor said, eyeing Chad. "Allow me to rephrase." He moved closer to Chad and whispered in his ear. "Tell me, young man, what did you stick in your dick?"

Here it comes, Chad thought. The hard part.

"It was, well, um . . ." It was time to spit it out. Not easy. A rod of pain shot through his middle, urging him on. "A piece of spaghetti," Chad finally said.

The intern's eyes looked huge, swollen. He hadn't noticed before, but he could now see her nipples through her shirt.

"You're kidding, right?" the doctor asked, a grin tugging at his lips shaming Chad, as if he needed shaming.

"Dead serious," Chad said, closing his eyes against the mirth he knew had to be coming.

The doctors turned to one another and smirked. Then the intern exited, leaving Dr. Tyberg to examine the damage. But the noodle had disappeared from view, so there was nothing to see.

"We'll need to call urology to retrieve the pasta," the doctor said. "It was uncooked I assume?"

Chad just nodded, and pulled the sheet over his head.

But he had to repeat the embarrassing tale yet again when finally he met his savior Dr. Muruve, the urologist on call. A kidney transplant specialist, Dr. Muruve had seen all manner of objects inserted into penises. He was surprised that so many people were unaware that the penis was a "one-way" organ.

Somehow, Chad made it through the story, ending up in the cystoscopy suite where a syringeful of anesthetic gel injected into his urethra delivered a brief respite from his agony. The gel was soon followed by a large cylindrical tube carrying a tiny camera on a hunt for the offending noodle. Dr. Muruve easily located the fragments of pasta, slightly more limp coming out than they were going in.

The rod finally free of his body, Chad left the hospital as fast as he could run. Of course, it was a story he'd forever keep to himself. Which is why his mother could never understand why, from then on, her son suddenly turned his nose up at every Italian dish she prepared.

PB AND SLAY

8

Dick, a sixty-eight-year-old retired glass worker, was always hungry. Early in their marriage, Dick's wife, Dora, marveled at her husband's ability to stay slim despite his love of food. As Dick aged, however, so did his metabolism. Out of nowhere, it seemed, Dick acquired a paunch. Throughout their thirty-five years together, Dora cooked all of Dick's meals and even prepared his snacks. She lived to serve her man.

Dick's other defining feature was his inability to sleep. Many times every night, he would wake, haul his big body out of bed and proceed to the bathroom or kitchen, or both.

In the midst of yet another restless sleep, Dick opened his eyes and cursed at the time: 3:11 a.m. His stomach rumbled and he let a loud one go under the covers. The stink prodded him out of bed. Standing too fast, he felt woozy. He stumbled, dizzy, to the closet, grabbed a robe from the hook and pulled it on. The frilly pink fabric ripped under the pressure of his bicep. Whoops, wrong one.

Eyes half shut, he made his way downstairs, grasping the banister so he wouldn't fall. He crept to the kitchen in the dark, feeling the wall for the switch. He flicked it up, but blinded by the light, he thumbed it back down. Squinting was easier. Still feeling slightly dizzy, he thought of calling his doctor to set up an appointment. Ever since he started those anti-hypertensive medications he didn't feel right. It seemed his episodes of dizziness were becoming more frequent and more prolonged.

Dick headed for the pantry. He opened the double doors but without his glasses on, he found it all fuzzy inside. He peered closer. Reaching for a jar of peanut butter, he surprised himself by knocking over a half dozen cans. He jumped out of the way, saving his toes, just before the cans fell to the floor, one at a time, with a clackety-clack. He bent over his stomach and replaced them, then carried his jar of Skippy to the kitchen island in the center of the room.

Ever since he was a child, Dick loved eating peanut butter from the jar with whatever utensil he found lying around. No cutlery? No problem. All he needed was a finger. Right beside the sink, a spoon rested in the cereal bowl he had used just three hours earlier. Rice Krispies still clung to its rim. Dick unscrewed the jar and dug in. Now this was going to be good.

He spooned straight into his mouth and swallowed. Then he started to gag. And soon, he was coughing and spitting, like a dog foaming at the mouth, in the sink.

When he could see straight, Dick stumbled to the wall and flicked on the lights. Whatever he had eaten, not only was it not peanut butter, it definitely was not food. He grabbed the jar and pulled it close to read the label. The first word he saw was POISON, the first image, a skull and crossbones. Not good. Now he knew what he had eaten. It was that glass-etching compound he had bought to create frosted glass for the front door.

The compound contained eighteen percent ammonium bifluoride and fifteen percent sodium bifluoride. He had no idea what those chemicals were but they tasted like bitter sand and he had to get them out of his system fast.

Dick hung over the sink, his fingers in his mouth, trying to force himself to retch. No luck.

Still in his paisley PJs, he screwed the cap back on the jar, found his car keys in the hall table drawer, and ran out into the cold. Poison, damn it. He could die if he didn't hurry.

Dick gunned the engine and raced to the nearest hospital, a fifteen-minute drive that felt like hours. Pain was shooting through his stomach from all directions. It felt like he had swallowed a bomb, and at any second, it might explode.

Running toward the emergency room doors, Dick was sweaty and light-headed. That's when his bowels opened in his pants. Wet and soiled, he kept moving. Time was ticking.

The security guard standing on duty outside the hospital entrance may not have been medically trained, but having worked in the emergency department for years, he sure could recognize someone in trouble. And in this case it wasn't hard. Forty yards from the entrance, Dick was on all fours, vomiting. The guard radioed for the triage nurse.

Within minutes, Dick was on a stretcher, being whisked inside the building. He was still clutching the jar. The nurse hooked up Dick to a heart rate monitor and attached a blood pressure cuff to check his vital signs.

"I thought it was peanut butter," he said to the doctors and nurses above him. "Peanut butter, I love peanut butter." He sounded deliriously happy, like a child on his birthday.

"Don't worry, Mr. Vitus," a young doctor soothed. He examined the contents on the jar's label.

"It says here exactly what you've ingested. You've poisoned yourself with fluoride. We've sent some blood samples to the lab, and we're placing a call to the Poison Control Center. We'll have you taken care of in no time. You're in the right place."

Dick started to shake. His muscles twitched. The nausea was heating up like a volcano. "My stomach!" he yelped. "Get me a bowl!"

"Poison Control Line 2," a nurse called.

"I just have to get the phone, Mr. Vitus. I'll be right back," the doctor said.

He turned to slide open the curtains draping the cubicle. Watching him leave, Dick sat up and tried to shout. He fell back against the bed with a thud. The monitor indicated asystole, telling the army of health care workers and support staff that rushed to his side that Dick's heart had stopped beating.

"Code blue, acute care 6, code blue, acute care 6," intoned overhead.

For the next forty-five minutes, hemodynamic and anti-arrhythmic drugs targeted Dick's collapsed veins. Amiodarone, lidocaine, bretylium, atropine, dopamine. Ampoule after ampoule exchanged hopeful hands. But to the shock of the emergency room staff, who were quite sure that nice Mr. Vitus would walk out of the hospital the next day, he was pronounced deceased at 4:45 a.m., as his wife still slept snug in their bed at home.

The autopsy, performed that afternoon, showed that Dick's esophagus and stomach were only moderately inflamed, and the remainder of the exam was normal. But a review of the blood tests taken just before he died told the story. Dick had suffered from severe hypocalcemia. His calcium level had dropped so low that it sparked a fatal heart rhythm.

Enormous amounts of fluoride ion had been dumped from Dick's stomach into his circulation. In a process known as chelation, the fluoride immediately attached itself to the calcium in Dick's bloodstream, irrevocably forming a calcium-fluoride complex. His postmortem fluoride level was 20 milligrams per liter, a hundred times the normal level.

Fluoride, a metabolic poison, is used to manufacture many industrial agents including aluminum, steel and glass. It is also found in fertilizers, roach powder and rat poison. The amount of fluoride that is added to toothpaste as sodium fluoride is tiny, at only about 1100 parts per million or about one milligram per gram of toothpaste. Poor Dick ate the equivalent of thousands and thousands of times what would be found on a typical toothbrush.

A case similar to Dick's took place in the early 1940s, when roach powder was mistaken for powdered milk in a prison cafeteria. The result? One simple error caused illness in 263 people and a whopping forty-three deaths.

BUZZ KILL

9

George was only five when his father first handed him a hammer. George's dad had been taught the love of carpentry by his own father, who had been taught by his. According to family lore, George had descended from the great woodworkers of Renaissance England; apparently, his forefathers had built Hampton Court Palace during the reign of Henry VIII. A distant uncle — so the story went — had been a master carver for the British fleet and was aboard the HMS *Victory* when Horatio Nelson was shot dead in the Battle of Trafalgar in 1805.

George was proud of his shop. He built pieces of furniture that he sold through a local merchant in town, just outside of Adelaide, in the state of South Australia. His specialty was oversized rustic dining tables. Over the years, George had established a stellar national reputation. He received orders for his work from all over the state. Building on his local fame, he aimed to expand his export business to countries all over the world.

Comfortable around power tools, George opened a shop that was home to a number of saws, including circular, band, chain and of course, see, which he built for the children he hoped one day to have. Still a bachelor at thirty-four, George was tired of being alone and he longed to find a woman who shared his love of rural life.

George's family wasn't all about wood. The farm produced some of the best tomatoes, pumpkins and melons in the state. George also had an apiarist license, which permitted the farm to engage in beekeeping. The Department of Primary Industries and Resources South Australia required all bee-keepers to be fully licensed.

In his youth, George had been stung so many times that he was now immune to the apitoxin that worker honeybees injected. Lately, though, George had noticed that the bees in his apiary seemed more likely to swarm and sting within a wider radius of the hives than was usual.

What could be causing all this aggression? George hoped that there were no Africanized honeybees infiltrating his hives. With a suspected parasite decimating bee populations all over the world, those crazy bees were the last things he needed.

One morning, George awoke with the sun. After rolling out of bed and brushing his teeth, he went straight to check on the hives, hoping his fears were born of paranoia. A quick scan and he was mollified. His bees were too busy polli-nating to sting. Bees trailed George as he strode to his shop, kicking up dust along the way. He flicked the pests away, but they kept returning, bouncing off his torso as he walked. They were threatening him, he knew. To protect their hives from intruders, bees bump first, and sting later. George was alarmed. If this came to a war, he was outnumbered. His only move would be to get rid of these hives and replace them.

Preparing for another relaxing day of sawing and banging, George donned his wraparound goggles then set to work on a light cherry wood dining table. It had been specially ordered by the wife of a successful winemaker from Coonawara. She had requested an oval top and legs carved like lions. It wouldn't have been his choice, but George would give the woman exactly what she wanted. The fact was, word of mouth garnered many more customers than advertising, and he was a businessman, after all.

The morning rays of sun snuck through the open windows of George's studio, making the sawdust-coated air shimmer. Woodchips flew around his workspace. The hook tooth blade of his Delta 1.5 horsepower industrial open stand band saw moved up and down, slicing wood like a knife through cheese.

George daydreamed. He was, perhaps, a little too comfortable around sharpened steel. He let his thoughts drift to Emma, a clerk at the Adelaide Arcade. He pictured her talking, looking down at the ground as she spoke. Somehow, George understood her. He was equally shy. It was time to ask her out for coffee, he knew, but having never dated before, the very thought paralyzed him.

The band saw jolted George out of his fantasy. It seemed that with every use, the blades made more noise.

Manufactured a decade earlier, the Delta was prone to mechanical problems. Its 1,725 rpm motor would frequently spark and bog despite the fact that it was fan-cooled. It was too loud and vibrated too much, and George knew it was time to either junk it, or replace the motor with a Baldor. He shook his head. Why would Delta fit an otherwise great machine with a crummy Emerson motor?

Sawing away, George thought about the last time a motor burnt out on his circular saw. He had taken the mess apart only to discover, hours later, that it had been running in the wrong direction. It took a whole day to rewire the motor, but first, he had spent hours searching the internet for instructions complete with diagrams.

Now, the room went slowly silent as the motor whined to a stop. It had stalled, damn it.

George was irritated, and the two cups of espresso he'd downed didn't help. Cursing under his breath, he suddenly felt a sting on his neck. He slapped, and caught the bee, squishing it against his skin. Take that.

To unstall the machine, George reached for the wood he had been feeding through the saw. At that moment, the rhythmic blade roared to life, and in an instant, sliced three fingers clean off his right hand. It happened so fast that George felt nothing as he stared agape at three small stumps, macabre pumping spigots of blood. George cried out and lurched backward, and the saw table followed, landing on top of his chest.

He stuck out his two-fingered right arm to right himself, and again touched the saw blade, as if it was controlled by a slasher in a horror movie. Panicked and flailing like a pig in a slaughterhouse, George screamed as his arm was nearly sawed off at the elbow.

Light-headed from blood loss but strangely experiencing no pain, he cried out again, and tried to push the saw and table off his torso with his left arm. The saw continued its rhythmic pulsation, though. Apparently more determined than George, its teeth struck the right side of his neck hitting his external and internal jugular veins before ripping through the carotid sheath and sinking deep inside his soft tissues and bone. Finally, the crunching died down as the band saw came to a halt on the concrete floor. The shop's floor was left littered with bloody fragments, including an indecipherable mix of bone and sawdust and various pieces of George.

A week later, the woman who had ordered her fashionable dining table sent her husband to pick it up. She had been unable to contact George on his cell phone but felt she had been more than patient. She had waited long enough.

Pulling a trolley behind him, the man entered the shop to find a horrid decomposing mess in the middle of the room. In the corner, he spotted the near-finished table. Clearly, there was nothing he could do for the poor man, but the fact was, the table was his and with a seventy-five percent down payment, he wasn't relinquishing it to the estate of the deceased. He loaded it onto the trolley and on the way out, swatted at the bees that were bouncing off of him. Then, once the table was safely stowed in the back of his truck, he pulled out his phone and called police.

BREAKFAST SPECIAL

10

It was just after noon on a Saturday when the first of the three friends awoke. It was an earlier than usual morning for these unemployed skateboarding slackers. With no job among them, their days were a blur of alcohol, Ecstasy and aimlessness.

Brian rose first and absently disengaged himself from the cold slice of pizza stuck to his forearm. Meat Lovers' Delight, yum. He bit into the rubbery cheese and left the scrap of crust on his bed. Then, picking his butt, he ambled half-dazed across the room toward the toilet.

"Yowch!" Jason whimpered as Brian accidentally tripped on his ankle. Then he moaned, rolled over, and curled back into a ball on the shag carpet where he slept.

By the time Brian's stream of urine found its way inside the toilet bowl, his bladder was nearly empty. Leaking urine through his shorts and down his right thigh, he cracked open one eye for just a moment. Retreating back to bed, he stomped on Jason's other ankle midway through his journey.

Lying on the recliner, clad in gray sweatpants and a drab T-shirt, Marty farted. A potent mix of last night's munchies, the gas rose and drifted like a toxic cloud before settling like a blanket over his buddies. Jason bolted upright. What 210 pounds of pressure on his ankles couldn't do, one of Marty's farts could. It was more effective than an alarm clock.

"I'm hungry," Jason mumbled. Foggy from a night of partying, he shuffled to the kitchen, ready to fry up a feast. Piles of dishes, along with an assortment of half-finished cans and empty bottles, littered counters. The green garbage bag was leaking brown goo onto the floor.

"There's nothin' to eat in this place," he grumbled as he searched for ingredients in the fridge. There was nothing he could whip up from bottles of barbecue sauce, vintage salad dressing, open cans of flat Diet Coke, a couple of slices of processed cheese, a stick of margarine, a bag of milk, two eggs, and a lime.

Hunting through the cupboards instead, he settled on a long forgotten box of pancake mix. Where did that come from? Was it there before he and the guys had moved in? By the time Jason began mixing milk, eggs and powder, his buddies had joined him in the kitchen. They swept wrappers from chairs and sat on stools, waiting to be served. Marty was hunched over the table, head in hands, nose dripping. He pinched it and wiped the mucous on his sweats. Mid-June. Hay fever.

His seasonal allergies and accompanying asthma were a lifelong affliction that Marty tried to ignore. Exposure to molds, cats and dogs caused his nose to dribble like an old man's penis after a midnight trip to the bathroom. At twenty, he had been living on the street and in friends' houses and apartments for the past four years. Marty earned his living holding his palm up on street corners or squeegying car windshields stopped at busy downtown intersections. A skinny pale kid, he was chronically fatigued with perpetual dark circles under his eyes. Add a scowl and many drivers were too fearful not to fork over their loose change.

"When are those pancakes ready, bro? I'm starved, man," Marty moaned. Between bits of a slice of hard yellow cheese, he took sips of a Diet Coke he had scored from the fridge.

"In five," Jason said.

Brian wandered over to the stove and sniffed. "Ugh! Smells like shit, man! What the hell are in those things?"

"I put shit in them," Jason said, barely moving his mouth. He dragged on his cigarette, the second of the young day. Snickering, he flicked the ashes into the mixture. After a few moments of trying to mold the pancake mix into circles in the frying pan, he gave up and just plopped down lumpy shapes.

The scraps Marty had scrounged from the kitchen barely dented his appetite. Just the smell of food cooking made his mouth water. A few minutes later, Jason dumped a pile of brown ill-shaped pancakes with burnt edges in the center of the table. Three sets of hands attacked them.

As half-chewed pulps spewed out of Jason's and Brian's mouths, Marty kept eating.

"What the hell are you doing?" he asked. "That's totally gross."

Brian was spitting the remnants on the table. "These taste awful! What the hell?" he yelled. "What did you do? Dip them in rubbing alcohol?"

Jason was already on his way to the sink to wash out his mouth.

"They're fine! Just quit puking on the table while I'm eating. And pass the syrup, would ya?" Marty said, half laughing.

Soon, though, Marty felt something crawling in the back of his throat. He tried to clear it, but it refused to budge. As he started heaving, his breath dammed as if it had nowhere to go. His face flushed hot, and his eyes filled with tears.

"Marty, you're lookin' sick, buddy," Jason said.

Marty stopped chewing. He needed that Ventolin inhaler he had used in the summers as a boy, but he hadn't seen it around in years. Feeling suddenly dizzy, he could hear his friends talking but their voices sounded far away. He opened his mouth but found that he couldn't form words. His last thought as he fell sideways to the floor was: "Syrup, where's the syrup?"

Watching their friend literally nosedive off the stool, Jason and Brian looked at each other. They almost burst out laughing but the sound of the rasps coming from Marty's throat shocked them into seriousness.

Jason bent down and flipped over his friend. "You okay, man?" he asked.

Marty's features were becoming blurred by the rapidly spreading swelling.

"Call an ambulance!" Jason shouted. He wasn't about to start CPR, figuring that whatever was hurting his friend was probably still on his lips and in his mouth.

In six short minutes, paramedics streamed into the apartment and descended on Marty's body, lying still on the dirty kitchen floor. His friends stood by, heads down, hands in pockets.

Having seen anaphylactic reactions many times, the medics leapt into action with intravenous lines, epinephrine, endotracheal tubes and oxygen. They knew full well that the body's rapid responses to agents such as peanuts, shellfish, drugs and insect bites could kill a person within seconds. They just hoped they had made it in time.

After twenty minutes of work, the medics found a pulse and transported Marty to hospital. But their efforts were wasted. Within hours of lying in a hospital bed, hooked up to machines that were supposed to be saving his life, Marty suffered a cardiac arrest from which he could not be resuscitated.

The coroner who performed the autopsy noted edema (swelling) of the pharynx and larynx. Marty's still lungs were hyperinflated, filled with mucus plugs. The cause of death was listed as an allergic reaction causing a blocked airway and cardiac arrest.

On the scene, the paramedics had listened to Marty's friends relate the sequence of events. They delivered the open box of pancake mix to the coroner who reviewed its contents, looking for evidence of the fatal pathogen.

The box, which had sat open on the pantry shelf, indicated that the mix had expired five years ago. A sample, sent to the Department of Environmental Health Services, showed that it contained excessive levels of mold, including fusarium, penicillium, aspergillus and mucor. As it turned out, mold was one of Marty's long-standing allergies. He had died from eating moldy pancakes. It was the last brunch the three friends would ever share.

FRIENDS AND ENEMAS

11

Usually gay and happy, Jamal arrived in the emergency room gay and in severe pain. Leaning on his lover, Chris, for support, Jamal was forced to stand at the triage desk. Sitting was, well, impossible.

"Tell me what happened," the nurse said. A questionnaire sheet sat on the desk in front of her. Jamal clutched his stomach. He was in too much pain to speak, and even if he wasn't, the story caused too much shame to relate out loud. What he didn't know was that Helen had been an emergency room nurse long enough to be immune to embarrassing stories.

Chris did the honors.

Helen listened. She kept a straight face as she concentrated on making neat checkmarks in the boxes on her sheet. When Chris finished speaking, she looked up at the men standing before her. It was late on a Saturday night, and Chris was wearing tight jeans, a muscle shirt, and a neon orange hard hat. Jamal was holding the back of a chair, refusing to sit.

"When did you say the abdominal pain started?" Helen asked no one in particular.

"About four hours later," Jamal moaned.

"And why did you do this again?" This was clearly the nuttiest story she had heard in all of her years of nursing. She had heard of strange sexual practices among gay men, and had seen some weird stuff, but nothing approached this.

"I'm not judging you boys. I just don't get the motivation," Helen said. She was curious.

"Like I said," Jamal answered even though he was saying it for the first time. "We were just fooling around." He added, as an excuse: "We were buzzed, you know?"

Helen didn't know. She wasn't the get-buzzed type.

"Your pulse is fast," Helen said. She wrapped a cuff around Jamal's upper arm. She inflated it by squeezing the rubber ball at the end of the tube. "Blood pressure's fine, though. I'll need to take your temperature, too," she added, then blushed. "Not rectally."

Chris chuckled, despite himself. Helen stuck the thermometer in Jamal's ear, then pulled it out.

"It's up," she noted. "Hold on, boys. I'll get a wheelchair."

Just the thought of sitting filled Jamal's eyes with tears. He turned to Chris.

"How in the world did I let you do it?" he asked him. "How did we let it get that far?"

Chris shrugged. He didn't know. In the heat of the moment,

you did things you would otherwise never consider. Besides, he stopped short of reminding his friend, it was Jamal's idea.

The nurse wheeled the chair toward the patient. Holding his middle with both hands, he just shook his head. "Can't sit," he reminded her.

Helen tried to guide him to the acute room but after a few shuffling steps, it was clear that Jamal would have to be carried.

Chris lifted his friend onto a gurney and, curled in a fetal position, Jamal let the wheels deliver him down the hall. He thought he could hear dozens of health care workers and support staff murmuring and giggling as he rolled past. Maybe he was paranoid, but it sure didn't seem like it. In fact, news of the patient's fiasco had already snaked its way around the emergency department.

The gurney took a detour to the radiology lab. Jamal waited for his turn in the hallway outside the X-ray room. The pain, initially spasmodic, was now constant and intense. The technician, a devout Muslim who considered homosexuality the behavior of deviants, opened the door and wheeled Jamal inside. She placed a flat metal plate under his back, asked him to hold his breath and clicked the camera in the direction of his stomach.

The emergency room doctor appeared within minutes, holding a clipboard. As Dr. Kiely began to read the notes in the chart, his eyes bugged behind fashionable wire-rimmed glasses. He scratched his head.

"Okay, Mr. Khan. Let's review this. What happened?"

Jamal's stomach hurt too much for him to feel the pain of shame anymore. It was time to get help, fast.

"We were just fooling around," he insisted.

"Okay," the doctor said. "Do you have any history of a psychiatric disturbance or have you ever seen a psychiatrist?"

"No," Jamal barked. He was curled on his side, and pain was erupting from his backside. Suddenly, he was at his breaking point. How were all these questions helping him? Couldn't they just get on with it so he could get out of this place?

"Just take it out or get someone to take it out!" he shouted with all the strength he could muster. "I'm in pain, for Christ's sake! I don't want to relive this anymore! I just want it behind me!"

Dr. Kiely almost smiled, but caught himself.

"Just a brief synopsis," he said. "And then we can figure out exactly how to help."

Jamal sighed then started to talk.

"My boyfriend and I, we were fooling around, we were kinda high, and we were role-playing. Since he's a construction worker, he thought it would be kinda fun to, you know, play construction worker, so he got on his outfit, tool belt, hard hat, the whole thing." The doctor glanced over at Chris. Evidently he didn't have time to change, he mused.

Jamal felt like his stomach was being slashed to shreds. Clutching it, he continued.

"We were, you know, fooling around, heating up, and after awhile, he thought he could spice things up some more — you know, take it to the next level. He told me he had a surprise in store for me. Next thing I know, he comes into the living room with a funnel and a bag of concrete mix. We were, you know, hot. We weren't really thinking."

The doctor listened, rapt. "Go on," he urged. He had stopped scribbling with his pen.

"I lay back, lifted my legs, put my feet against the wall. Chris, well, he stuck the funnel in my ass with a bit of lube and after mixing the concrete — he's a construction worker you know — he poured it in pretty deep. It felt amazing at first, I just flipped, and really, we had the best time. It was almost worth it. But then, after a few hours, well, it started to ache. We tried to get it out all sorts of ways, but when the cramps became unbearable, he brought me here. The pain is really killing me, Doc!" Jamal was relieved to have it all out there in the open. He grimaced, started to sweat.

Dr. Kiely performed a quick examination. Was there a hard mass in the lower abdomen? He wasn't quite sure. He had seen lots of foreign bodies inside the rectum — a stick, a cucumber, a yo-yo. He had never seen a gerbil, although that was the question everyone seemed to ask. This was the first time he had seen anyone intentionally use their colon as a concrete mixer.

"Well, Mr. Khan, obviously we have to find a way to get the concrete out," the doctor said. "I'm thinking a gastroenterologist or surgeon, but give me a couple of minutes to decide who would be right for the job."

Dr. Kiely rested his chin in his hand as he looked at the X-ray. In Jamal's lower intestine there sat a whitish blob of what he now knew was hardened concrete. At the top of the mass, though, there was something else visible. It looked like the cherry atop a vanilla sundae. He scratched his head not for the first time that night.

The doctor returned to his patient and leaned over the stretcher's metal railing. "Well, Mr. Khan, the general surgeon is on his way. We're going to have to operate."

"Just get it out, get it out, get it out," Jamal whimpered, his tears now soaking the sheets.

Less than an hour later, the surgeon dilated Jamal's anus and safely delivered a two-pound mass of concrete. Using a chisel, he was able to separate the cherry-like object hiding inside the concrete at the top of the mass. It was, of all things, a Ping-Pong ball.

The following morning, Jamal was released from the hospital. On his way out, he refused psychiatric counseling. What the hell do doctors know about sex, anyway? he wondered, imagining Dr. Kiely and the prim nurse assuming the boring, old missionary position. Little did Jamal know, however, that he suffered from a condition known as klismaphilia, which would inevitably lead him back to the hospital for future anal extractions.

Klismaphilia refers to sexual gratification achieved with enemas, in this case a concrete one. People who have this condition enjoy the stimulation of nerve receptors within the anus and rectum, often because their mothers or nurses gave them frequent enemas during childhood.

In this case, the patient's lover likely inserted the Ping-Pong ball after the concrete, to act as a plug. That's because klismaphiliacs try to retain their enemas, and therefore their pleasure, for as long as possible. As the concrete hardened, it released heat, which propelled the ball to the front of the line. The warmth of the reaction exacerbated Jamal's pleasure, but sadly for him, that pleasure was soon eclipsed by its evil twin: pain.

HOT STUFF

12

Coffee, like all caffeinated beverages, is a liquid drug. The more you drink, the more you need. Hundreds of millions of consumers spend billions of dollars on coffee and its middle-class relatives — tea, Coke and chocolate. More than half of all North Americans down their beloved coffee every single day.

Lori loved a good drink, lots of them in fact, but her poison was a lot harder than coffee. She spent her weekends gulping alcohol shots — tequila, vodka, Scotch — whatever she could wrangle out of the men who were hanging around the cocktail bars in downtown Dallas, hoping to score. But as soon as her drink was down, Lori would flash a smile, and move on.

At around 6 p.m. on Friday night, Lori would start getting dressed for a night on the town. She would choose her ensemble from the inside out — starting with her lacy thong and matching bra, then wriggling her way into a tube top, tight skirt and, of course, stilettos.

After a night of knocking back rounds and making the rounds, Lori was too drunk to know that it was near closing time at Taste of Asia karaoke bar. Tilted on a stool, she gripped the bar for balance. Her makeup, so carefully applied in her bathroom mirror with the fluorescent lighting, now looked more like The Joker than the Lady Gaga look she sported when she entered. Her lids kept drooping.

"Crap. What time is it? I've got work tomorrow," she said, slurring to her roommate Bev, her responsible friend.

Every girl needed a Beverley, Lori always thought when she'd wake up hungover with no memory of her trip home from the bar, let alone how she got into her nightie and into bed.

Tonight, Bev sat beside her friend, sipping her Fresca with lime through a straw, and answering emails on her iPhone. Unlike Lori, Bev was wearing jeans and a simple white blouse. What she didn't know was that her horn-rimmed glasses excited some men even more than Lori's cleavage and tiny skirts.

Bev checked her phone for the time. "It's nearly two!" she shouted over the pounding rhythmic bass. "What time do you start tomorrow?"

Lori was too wasted to follow the simplest conversation. And yet she wasn't too far gone to drink. She sat up straight, stuck out her chest, and scanned the room for another sucker. Even with the messy makeup, she made quick eye contact with a pack of men smoking at the end of the bar, and within seconds, they huddled around her, fighting to offer a light.

Beverley slipped her phone into her purse and sighed. She'd missed her opening. Now she'd have to battle the crowd.

"Sorry boys," she said, pushing her way into the circle. "It's closing time and trust me, you wouldn't enjoy it if you could get it."

Lifting Lori under her arms, she dragged her from the bar stool and led her toward the exit. Outside, the freezing night air slapped Lori's bare shoulders and legs. But her skin felt warm, numb.

"Wher we gon?" she slurred, flopping like a dead fish onto her friend.

"Night's over, baby. You're punching cash tomorrow bright and early, remember?"

With one hand circling her friend's waist, Bev used the other to wave for a taxi. It took ten minutes before a cab finally screeched to a stop in front of the women. By then, both were about to tip over, Lori from the weight of alcohol loosening her limbs, and Bev from Lori's body weight.

After directing her friend into the cab, Bev jumped in and slammed the door. She fastened both of their seat belts as the driver sped into the night.

"You need coffee, hon," Beverley said, brushing the hair from Lori's face. Her friend was drooling onto her tube top.

"Stop over there, please," Bev said, motioning the driver to a twenty-four-hour coffee shop up ahead. The car pulled up in front of the gas station pumps. Beverley opened the door.

"Wait here. I'll be right back," she said, leaving Lori slumped across the back seat.

"She better not throw up in my car," the driver said in some mysterious accent Beverley could hardly make out.

"Don't worry," Bev said. "That's not her style."

Bill had worked at Overtime Coffee for two decades now. It was in a prime spot, just outside the entertainment district. Every weekend, just after 2 a.m., he could expect the same scene: carloads of drunks swarming the place for coffee to perk them up before they headed home to bed. Some would loiter in the booths while others preferred to take off fast, their liquid drug sealed inside a recyclable cup. For some, the shop had become a post-party pickup joint for the second string players who had failed to hook up during regulation time. Overtime indeed.

A fresh pot of coffee was boiling and dripping onto the burner.

"I'll take two Larges to go, please," Beverley said.

"Coming up," said Bill, filling two cups. He placed them, steaming, on the counter. "Careful," he said before stating the obvious. "They're hot."

In exchange, Beverley handed the man three dollars. She covered the cups with plastic lids. Even with her leather gloves on, they were almost too hot to handle. She carried the coffee to the cab and placed one on the roof while she opened the back door.

"Lori!" she yelled in her friend's ear to rouse her from the seat. "Time to get up!"

"Sssshhhh! Im finsla aseplpa," Lori mumbled.

Beverley grabbed her arm and yanked her to sitting. "Here ya go, hon. Hot coffee. It'll help. Be careful, though," she said, handing her the cup.

Beverley remembered to rescue her own cup from the cab roof before sliding in beside her friend and slamming the door. She gave the driver the address and sighed. Time to go home.

The cab jerked forward and then Lori screamed so loud, the windows threatened to shatter. Startled, Beverley tipped her coffee and it splashed onto the seat, hitting her knee on the way down.

"AAAAHHHHHHH!" she screamed too, creating a chorus that made the driver slam the brakes and pull over.

In the back, Beverley was madly brushing the coffee from her scalded leg and grabbing Lori's cup at the same time. The driver turned and she thrust both cups at him.

"Take these and drive to a hospital! Now!" she cried.

Cradling her friend in her lap, Beverley watched Lori gasp for breath. Suddenly, she began to cough drops of blood that splattered onto the back of the driver's seat.

"Lori! Stay awake!" Bev shouted, but her friend just moaned.

The cabbie sped to the hospital. All he had needed was one last fare for the night and somehow he had ended up with two drunk lesbians, a car full of coffee and blood and chances were, a stiffed fare. Maybe he could boot them out here, on the street. But what if the coughing one died. Then he'd be up shit's creek.

"Thirty dollars please," he said, as he swung to a stop at the emergency room sign.

To his surprise, Beverley opened her purse and handed him two $20 bills before kicking open the door and yelling like a crazy lady for help.

Within minutes, an orderly was helping her drag a barely conscious Lori into the hospital where they were directed toward the acute room. The charge nurse summoned Dr. Robles. He immediately ordered an intubation tray.

Lori was struggling with each loud breath, shooting spits of blood onto the sheets. Her heart was racing and her blood pressure had dropped. The nurse hooked her up to an IV.

"What happened?" asked Dr. Robles. Around him swarmed doctors in greens.

Beverley, standing in the room's shadows, stepped forward. She cleared her throat then began.

"She was so drunk, I thought we had to stop for coffee. But just after I handed her the cup, as I was fastening my seat belt, she screamed, and when I turned to look, I saw that her cup was empty. The coffee was gone. It was scalding. I know because I spilled some on my leg. It was scalding and I think she drank it all in one big gulp. She started choking!"

Dr. Robles attached a pouch containing a milky white liquid to Lori's IV. It was 50 milligrams of Diprivan, or Propofol, also now known as "the Michael Jackson drug," the stuff that killed the superstar in the comfort of his home. As M.J. never learned, the hypnotic medicine should be administered only by trained anesthetists in hospital or clinic settings with full resuscitation equipment available. Administering Propofol at home is like giving yourself chemotherapy or removing your own appendix.

Examining Lori's mouth, the doctor saw that her throat was red and swollen. Intubating her, he established an airway through which she could breathe. But despite his efforts, her blood pressure plummeted. To maintain it, he established a right internal jugular central venous line and added intravenous Dopamine as well as liters of saline to her IV.

In the ICU, Lori lay unconscious overnight. The next day, her mouth started bleeding and it was impossible to stem the flow. The young woman was hemorrhaging. The doctor ordered units of blood, providing initial stability. A gastroenterologist was summoned to perform a scope of her esophagus and stomach.

"It's always a bit easier when they're sedated and intubated," Dr. Stotland explained to the resident assisting. He maneuvered the scope and its camera around the endotracheal tube and was immediately met with profound swelling. Close to aborting the procedure, he squeezed around the swollen tissue and passed the long black snake-like tube into the esophagus.

"I've never seen anything like this," he said, amazed.

Bright red, friable and bleeding, Lori's esophagus was a cylindrical tube of burnt tissue. There was nothing to repair.

"She has a massive third degree thermal injury to her esophagus," Dr. Stotland said to the resident as he snapped off his gloves after the procedure. "The entire esophagus must be removed. There's nothing else we can do."

But there was no time. Blood spouted from Lori's esophagus into her nasogastric tube. She was suffering from hematemesis. Despite the doctors' attempts to pump dozens of units of blood, platelets and plasma into her system, she died from massive blood loss secondary to diffuse esophageal bleeding from a liquid burn. The coffee, meant to wake her, had ultimately put her to sleep.

HAIR TODAY GONE TOMORROW

13

It was Miranda's fourth hospitalization in six months. At twenty-two years of age, she had lived with Crohn's disease for almost half of her life. Crohn's, like its cousin ulcerative colitis, is an inflammatory bowel disease, known simply as IBD, a condition in which the body mistakes the cells of the bowel wall for foreign invaders and goes on the attack. The unfortunate result of this misfire is intestinal swelling, mucous, bleeding, gas and pain.

For the luckiest of sufferers, IBD is mild. But for Miranda, the condition was severe and although she tried to cope, it was, frankly, bumming her out. The last four years were a haze of drugs and sex, interrupted only by her frequent rushes to the toilet and sometimes the hospital.

During adolescence, Miranda underwent multiple surgeries

to resect parts of her inflamed intestines but the Crohn's stood firm. Losing the battle, she started drowning in fear and depression. As a teen, she was sometimes so low that she often packed a sack and hitched rides out of town, just to get away. Her parents got used to calling the local police, who had come to know Miranda and her frequent exits. Sadly, her moodiness and attention-seeking behavior only intensified as she grew.

Miranda lay in yet another hospital bed. The scene was so familiar — the bed that creaked when she turned, the cardboard pillow, the stench of urine mingling with disinfectant — she felt like she was in her second home. It was the third week of another hospitalization, and here she lay, hooked up to IV again. Her stack of magazines lay read and reread on the bedside table. She sighed. There was no end in sight.

In order to give her overactive bowels a rest, Miranda was denied food and drink. In place of oral nutrition, liquid nutrients called total parenteral nutrition, or TPN, entered her body through an intravenous line piercing her subclavian vein, just beneath her left clavicle. Miranda watched as round-the-clock nurses hung bags of yellow, white or clear liquids that emptied as fat globules into her body. Broken down into the bare nutritional essentials, the liquid food bypassed her bowels so there was no need for enzymes, digestion and absorption. Miranda got ready for the cramps. They came in spasms and got worse in the afternoon.

She pressed the call button.

A voice came through the intercom static into her room. "Can I help you?"

"I need my pain meds, please," Miranda said, looking

forward to the drug sweeping away the pain and sliding her into relief.

"I'll send in your nurse."

Soon, middle-aged Maggie — who must be somebody's Nana, Miranda thought — ambled into the room. She looked at Miranda with kind eyes.

"Sorry, hon," Maggie said. "You're not due for two hours."

"But I'm in pain. I'm cramping again. I'm dying here."

"It's only been an hour, love. Should I call Dr. Hower?"

Here we go again, Nurse Maggie thought. With this girl, it was the same routine, over and over. The notes said codeine every four hours, but Miranda tried to get it every two. Maggie shook her head, but the girl was persistent. You could say that about her.

"Your anti-inflammatories are right here," the nurse said, dropping two pills and a small cup of water on Miranda's nightstand. "Maybe these will help."

When Miranda could no longer hear the nurse's footsteps in the hall, she pulled open the nightstand drawer. At the back, in a small jewelry pouch, lay her secret stash. She shook the pouch until a pill fell into her hand. She popped it into her mouth and washed it down, for the third time this morning, with water. It was Temazepam, a drug that was supposed to reduce her anxiety but clearly wasn't doing its job.

Miranda eyed the white bag of fluid hanging from a silver intravenous pole, and followed its milky trail as it dripped through the tube. The image flickered off and on as she fought to focus. Her vision was a blur, and she drifted into a blackened sleep.

Miranda was awakened by cramps ripping apart her belly. She pulled herself out of sleep and swung her feet to the floor. Taking her shampoo and conditioner along, she rolled her IV pole down the hall to the bathroom.

Once there, she closed and locked the door. Then she disrobed, marveling at herself in the mirror. Now that was one skinny dame. Her mother always said it and it was true: you could never be too rich or too thin.

Miranda stepped into the shower, letting the spray warm her skin. She washed and conditioned her hair, not noticing as wet clumps slid from her scalp to the shower floor. She did notice, however, just how similar the hair conditioner looked to the white liquid that emptied from her IV bag into her vein.

Her shower done, Miranda stepped out, toweled herself and made her way back down the hall.

Three weeks ago, along this same journey back to her room, Miranda had noticed a nurse's cart, temporarily abandoned in the hallway. On it sat medical instruments of all shapes and sizes. Miranda had spotted a 10 cc syringe, thinking it might come in handy during her stay, particularly if she wasn't being given the drugs she needed as fast as she needed them. So she had been sneaky. She had pinched the syringe off the cart and kept walking.

Now safely back on her bed, Miranda was pissed off. If the nurses weren't going to give her the drugs she needed, then she would make them. If she could just get their attention, make them see that she was really sick, then maybe they would give her the codeine now. It was worth a shot.

Miranda reached into the nightstand drawer for the

syringe, and aspirated it full of white liquid. Hearing voices, she jumped off the bed and checked up and down the hall. Then she ducked back into her room and injected the contents of the syringe into the clear plastic tubing connected to her torso.

"Did you hear that thump?" Maggie asked the nurse next to her before rising from her chair.

Maggie followed the sound to Miranda's room.

The first thing she saw was what appeared to be a child's hand reaching into the hallway. It was Miranda, sprawled on the floor, all eighty-eight pounds of her, next to a full syringe of what appeared to be her liquid nutrition.

"Call the doctor!" Maggie screamed, falling to Miranda's side. "Call a code! I can't get a pulse!"

Trained in the art of CPR, Maggie breathed air into Miranda's tiny body as her colleague rhythmically pumped on the girl's chest. Within minutes, a crash cart rolled in from the intensive care unit.

Youth was on Miranda's side, giving her a good chance at resuscitation. The emergency team was determined, trying for more than one hour to breathe life into the woman's dying lungs. But Miranda's body was so frail. Eventually, all of the pushing caused her ribs to crack. If the team had an inkling of what had transpired in the patient's room when she was alone, they may have been able to save her.

In searching for the cause of Miranda's sudden death, the autopsy focused on her chest and abdomen. The pathologist, Dr. Patrick, was a bald man with a belly that couldn't be contained by his belt. At first, he saw no obvious explanation for the young lady's demise. It was a mystery indeed. She was skeletal, yes, and her abdomen was a crisscross of scars both inside and out, but he knew the colitis was still active, because her bowel was inflamed.

The next day, while eating the salad his wife had packed to help him shed a few pounds, the doctor sat at his desk reviewing the previous day's slides through the giant eyes of his microscope. Teeny slices of lung tissue stared back at him. That's when he noticed something odd.

The tissue appeared normal. But the small arteries inside were not filled with blood. There was some material he did not recognize. Knowing a syringe had been found at the scene, Dr. Patrick matched its contents to the microscopic material on the slide. Bingo. The girl had been killed by hair conditioner that she, for some unknown reason, had injected into her intravenous line. The viscous material got no farther than the blood vessels of her lungs. The "hair conditioner embolus" had blocked the girl's blood vessels, immediately causing her death.

An embolism refers to the blockage of any blood vessel of the body by material, usually a blood clot. A pulmonary embolus is almost always due to a blood clot that forms in the legs and breaks off toward the heart. The heart pushes the clot into the lungs where it obstructs blood flow causing chest pain, shortness of breath, and if the clot is large enough, death.

Most intentional deaths from injection are due to drugs. While there have been reports of suicides resulting from the injection of unusual substances, such as snake venom, this is the only case of death by hair conditioner. And although reckless, the death was unintentionally caused by the patient's attention-seeking behavior. Sadly for Miranda, there would be no more showering of attention on her ever again.

ALIEN

14

Aminata was soaping up in the shower when she felt the lump. It didn't hurt but it was round and hard and there was no mistaking it. She rinsed, toweled, and dressed fast. A quick call to the nearest medical clinic and she was in the car, on her way.

A decade ago, Aminata Ndoye had immigrated to Canada from Senegal. She had only been hospitalized once before, and that was ages back. At that time, she was suffering from a severe foot infection that required intravenous antibiotics and a one-week stay at the Hôpital Aristide le Dantec in Dakar, the country's capital.

After that experience, Aminata had avoided doctors, scared that at regular checkups, they would find something wrong. In this country, she had yet to seek medical attention — until now. A three-hour wait behind her, Aminata was gowned and sitting on an exam bed explaining that she had found a lump. The doctor listened then asked Aminata to disrobe from the waist up.

Dr. Medinsis felt Aminata's left breast. There it was: an irregular mass in the upper right quadrant.

"When did you first notice this?" the doctor asked, unable to mask surprise.

"Just now. I felt it in the shower."

Concerned about the possibility of progressive and aggressive breast cancer, Dr. Medinsis had her secretary arrange an urgent mammogram for the following day.

"Come back in two days and we'll discuss the results," she told Aminata, touching her shoulder in an attempt to reassure her. "I should be able to get a verbal report from the radiologist just after you have the test."

Aminata arrived early, and tired, for her 11 a.m. appointment. She had been unable to eat or sleep the day before. This was her first mammogram and just the word sounded frightening.

The blonde technician directed her to the machine. She opened Aminata's gown and placed her breast between two metal plates. Aminata held her breath as the plates sandwiched her breast to spread it evenly and reduce the thickness of its tissue. The digital image entered the queue. The radiology clinic tried to ensure that all tests were interpreted within twenty-four hours, recognizing the rush of anxiety that most women experience awaiting results.

At first, the radiologist was sure that there had been a technical error. The results before him on the PACS digital system showed a startling abnormality the likes of which he had never seen. There was a calcified squiggly mass in the patient's left breast.

After an hour of poring over radiology and mammography texts and scanning the internet, Dr. Vickar still had no idea what he was looking at. Working at a large academic hospital, he was fortunate that two other radiologists possessed similar expertise in mammography. He called both to his work station and asked them to review the films. This was no technical error, the doctors all agreed. Staring at the strange images, they scratched their heads.

"She's from Africa, so this has to be something infectious," Dr. Vickar concluded. "Call one of our infectious disease guys. Maybe they can sort this out."

Soon, Dr. Leonay, the on-call infectious disease expert, was listening to the woman's history while cocking his head at the unusual mammogram. It took only seconds for him to make a diagnosis.

"Guinea worm," he said. "It's a parasitic condition. Also called Dracunculiasis. It's caused by a nematode or roundworm. You're looking at a dead male parasite that has lodged in her breast."

The other doctors were amazed. This man's medical knowledge, acquired through a two-year fellowship in parasitology in Ghana, was nothing short of encyclopedic.

"Gross," said Dr. Vickar, lost in the image. "Totally gross."

When he could drag his eyes away, Dr. Vickar called Aminata's referring doctor who struggled to understand what he was saying.

"It's Dracunculiasis," Dr. Vickar explained, sounding like he had dredged up the word from some old horror story.

When he heard only silence on the line, he continued. "You should probably just look it up so you can explain it to the patient. Either that, or refer her to our infectious disease guy, Dr. Leonay. It's your choice. But in the meantime, you can reassure her that she's not dying of cancer. What she's got may frighten her, though. It's a dead, calcified male parasitic worm embedded in her breast."

The description left Aminata's doctor recalling scenes from the film *Alien*. What she didn't know is that in fact, Dracunculiasis is a well-known disease in some parts of the world. In Africa, millions of people are infected as a result of drinking stagnant, contaminated water.

Unbeknownst to those unfortunate enough to acquire Dracunculiasis, the illness-causing water contains microscopic copepods, or water fleas, that play host to immature larvae of the guinea worm. Inside the fleas, the larvae grow for about two weeks, waiting for a victim to swallow them. Without a host to feed on, the larvae die. So without people, there would be no guinea worm population.

After the innocent victim drinks contaminated water, her stomach acid digests the hapless water fleas, but not the nematode larvae. Instead, the undigested larvae burrow through the small intestine into the abdominal cavity where they live at a parasite hotel, growing unrecognized by their human host. About three months later, having aged into adult worms, the male and female enjoy a night of parasite sex.

By now, the female worm may be as thick as a spaghetti

noodle and up to three feet long and still, the host human has no inkling of its presence. But the male worm does. Like a black widow or praying mantis, the male nematode dies (happily) after sex only to be absorbed by the body or become calcified. Only rarely, as was the case with Aminata, does the dead worm migrate to find a home in another part of the body.

It is only the female worm that tries to escape, and not for at least a year after entering the victim. Burrowing through tissue, the female creates a blister, usually in the lower limbs, and emerges from the wound. The attempted exit results in severe pain and burning, which the victim attempts to alleviate by immersing the leg in stagnant water. And thus the cycle continues. Into the water, the female releases hundreds of thousands of larvae, which are eaten by the water fleas waiting to infect another human.

As the worm emerges, Africans do what has been done for thousands of years: wrap the live worm around a small stick to remove it. The process causes weeks of painful burning and may cause secondary bacterial infections, which can recur because they do not produce immunity.

Dracunculiasis, also known as the fiery serpent, comes from the Latin phrase *affliction with little dragons,* a testament to the severe burning that a live alien worm causes on its way out. Amazingly, the disease was first chronicled over 3,000 years ago and is still alive and well.

THE MAN WHO LOST HIS HEAD

15

Betty, a passing motorist, found him. She saw roadkill in the middle of her lane — it could be a poor squirrel with a broken leg, she thought — so she did the Christian thing. She hit her flicker and pulled over.

He was lying facedown on the road. At least his head was facedown — although a gust of wind could have rolled it over. No matter what Islamic terrorists or drug lords say, heads and bodies should always be attached, Betty thought.

Standing above the dead stranger in her best Sunday dress and straw hat, Betty worried she might get hit by a car speeding too fast, its owner jabbering away on a cell phone. She thought she could see further trouble about a half mile up the road, but she had missed her eye doctor appointment last year, and her glasses were due for a prescription upgrade.

There was no doubt about it, though. This was clearly the back of a human head. Betty squatted, bending her knees, so as not to hurt her back, and peered at the man's profile. Nice looking, she thought. But he could sure use a shave.

Raised in a traditional Baptist home, Betty hadn't missed a Sunday service in seventy years. It was a half hour drive to the community church in Colby, Kansas, the closest town to her fourteen-acre farm.

She had been on her way to ride the pews when she stopped. It was darn lucky that she never drove more than twenty miles per hour — despite the frustration of anyone unfortunate enough to be stuck behind her on the two-lane road to church. Now, her beloved 65 AMC American Rambler, her first and only car, parked safely at the side of the road, blinked its hazards to warn those speeders to slow the heck down.

She opened her purse and pulled out her BlackBerry Torch. Should she dial 911, text or email for help?

"911. What's your emergency?"

"This is Betty Dawkins," she said, careful to enunciate clearly. "I'm along Interstate 70 headed west, about two miles outside of Colby and there's a head on the road. Darndest thing I ever did see. Looks like it came clean off the neck. Better tell Jed to get on down here," she said, then clicked End. Well, that was easy.

Betty dropped her trusty BlackBerry into her purse and grabbed the Glock from its Predator holster. She knew it was illegal to carry a concealed handgun in Kansas, but living on a farm for fifty-three years had a way of stirring up some fine rural-flavored paranoia.

Betty crouched over the man's head and stood guard. She looked up at the sky, prepared to shoot any circling buzzards, and then gazed down the road in case she had to use the gun to slow a car.

Minutes later, Betty's son, Sheriff Jed Dawkins, swerved his siren-blaring, light-flashing car to a stop, blocking the road. He jumped out, his own Glock in plain view in the holster on his hip.

Jed whistled long and loud through his teeth. "Okay, Ma, spill," he said. "What'd you do?"

"Well, son, I was driving to church and I seen what I thought was a squirrel maybe. I figured it was injured and I'd do something — not sure what. But as you can see, it ain't no squirrel unless it's a squirrel shaped like a head with a mustache."

The day was hot, the sun climbing high. Without wind, the head wasn't budging. Jed crouched to get a better look.

"That's a mighty bushy beard," he said. "Dang! I didn't think we had terrorists in these parts quite yet." He scratched his own head. "Betcha it's them drug gangs from the South. Heard they've moved up to Topeka. I got it from here Ma. Best you get goin' to church and pray for this fella."

Betty was torn between missing church for the first time in her life and staying right here, where the action was. She clucked, weighing the pros and cons. In the end, she didn't want God to punish her. Lord knows the farm needed rain.

"Give your mama a hug," Betty told her son, and he did as he was told. Then she climbed into her car, slammed the door, and pulled on her seat belt. She hit her flicker before carefully navigating the Rambler around the police car and honking Jed a goodbye. He was such a fine young man. And so handsome.

Half a mile up the road, Betty spotted a silver 1978 Corvette that had smashed into a group of Norway spruce. She slowed down but kept moving. She was late enough for church as it was. Instead, she committed a no-no, pulling her BlackBerry from her purse while driving. She pressed the first button on her speed dial.

"Jed," she said when he picked up. "There's a wrecked car up ahead. Figured you'd see it, son, but just wanted to give you the heads up. Don't forget, suppertime is at four. Sharp. I'm makin' possum."

Jed returned to his car, and called in the crash. His deputy was on the way. Mmm, possum, he thought, as he surveyed the head on the road.

Jed was careful to look, not touch, since the photographer wasn't yet on the scene. He pulled out his notepad and started scratching details. White male. Shoulder-length black hair. No shoulders. Eyes open, mouth closed. His skin was the pale hue one would expect when bloodless. His head looked like it had been made in a special effects studio.

Jed could see that the decapitation was quite clean. It looked as if the head had simply fallen off its neck.

Leaving his squad car to alert traffic, Jed scanned the roadside with his flashlight and caught a glimpse of something unusual. A thick rope was wrapped around the trunk of a large cottonwood tree, aka a *Populus deltoides*. He looked up, expecting a noose, but saw nothing dangling from its upper branches. Searching the brush for the end of the rope, he followed its coils and found its bloodied end, knotted in a circle.

Yowza. This scene was getting much more interesting all of a sudden.

The sound of sirens approached, and then there was Phil, Jed's deputy, by his side. He showed Phil the rope, told him his theory, then left him to man the head.

It was a short drive to the wreck. Although still recognizable, the Corvette's front end was crushed from what was obviously a head-on collision. Splinters from a mangled spruce tree were everywhere.

Jed walked to the driver's side, gun drawn. He'd been blindsided before. He had to be on guard.

The window had either been rolled down or shattered. With so much glass from the smashed windshield, it was impossible to tell. On the driver's side, there sat a body, strapped in, headless. Dressed in a white shirt drenched in blood, the man looked perfectly normal if you ignored the absence of his head, Jed thought. He had been right; it was a nice, clean decapitation.

He rummaged through the man's jean pockets, and came up with a wallet and a folded Home Depot receipt for $9.95. The word "Rope" was printed in purple ink.

Jed got into his car and returned to the head. Standing over it, he had a strange urge to kick the thing, see if it bounced or skidded on the road. It was a gruesome thought, he knew. But in this job, you had them all the time. It was all in a day's work.

He tilted up his hat then placed his hands squarely on his hips. Phil, who had been busy erecting pylons on the road, joined him. Both wore sunglasses so dark, their eyes seemed to vanish behind them.

"Suicide," he said to Phil, who nodded.

Jed expected that a quick phone call would confirm his theory. Likely, the guy had a long history of depression, or maybe drug abuse. Maybe he got caught in bed with the kids' babysitter and his wife was leaving him to rot. Maybe he'd been fired from the only job he'd ever held, or his life of poker had finally sucked his bank account dry.

Whatever the reason, Maxwell Hillayee, whose driver's license photo showed a happy enough looking fellow, was one methodical son of a bitch. He had purchased a ball of heavy-duty rope and picked a lonely stretch of road. And early on a Sunday morning, when there was no chance of being saved, he tied a triple-loop knot around the trunk of a poor, unsuspecting cottonwood tree. Maxwell must have gotten into his car, opened the window and then knotted the other end around his neck. Then he must have rammed the pedal of the L-48 185 horsepower engine right down to the floor.

The car was capable of zero to sixty miles per hour in 6.6 seconds, but the rope wasn't long enough to last. The tug was so sudden and so hard that Max's head flew through the window and landed at its final resting place, smack in the middle of the road. The Corvette, driven by a headless body, crashed into the trees where the rest of the man was laid to rest.

It wasn't rocket science, Jed thought, chewing on a blade of dead grass, tasting possum already. It was all in an honest day's work.

SQUISH KEBOBS

16

Just after midnight, Luigi raced along the Strada Statale highway in his Alfa Romeo 156, passing cars at speeds of 175 kilometers per hour. A gift from his father, the red sports car had a diesel-powered 2387 cc five-cylinder turbo engine that was controlled by a six-speed gearbox. Other cars were fast, yes. But they could eat his dust, Luigi thought.

After just days of practice, Luigi was expert at shifting gears. Enveloped by a leather magnesium frame driver's seat, he imagined himself at the Imola racetrack on the World Touring Car Championship. He could see the checkered flag beckoning and hear the crowd cheering him on. Whereas his friends grew up in soccer gear dreaming of kicking the winning goal in the World Cup final, Luigi spent his youth fantasizing about racetracks.

In the back seat, his childhood friends, Marco and Francesco, sat bolt upright, their hands balled in fists, knuckles white. They were pretending to be excited but strapped in on what felt like an amusement ride, they were praying for it to end. The speed was too far out of their control.

Marco wished he had stayed back when the phone rang. It was night, and he had final exams next week. But Luigi had heaped on the peer pressure, convincing him he'd have a blast. Now, Marco was regretting his weakness. He just wanted to make it back to school alive.

Stefano, Luigi's brother, had the misfortune of sitting in the passenger seat. Stoned and silent, Stefano stared through bloodshot eyes out the window at the blurred landscape as the car shot down the road like a projectile. Unlike his brother, Luigi preferred to race his car straight, free of the effects of drugs and alcohol.

As he tore through the SS highway, Luigi conquered each dimly lit curve. The silence, save for the sound of the engine's hum and the scream of tires, was nothing short of exhilarating. At sixteen, he felt like he was inside his very own video game. Like all teenagers, Luigi felt invincible, his body shockproof. That is, until he swung around a curve fifty miles faster than the design of the road allowed. Even Mario Andretti would have lost control at that instant, but he, of course, would have known better than to take the curve so quickly.

The Alfa Romeo careened left and right as Luigi lost control of the steering wheel before slamming into a chain-link fence surrounding an industrial complex. The car roared, and dragging parts of fence, it bounced over knolls and skidded, coming to rest a hundred yards from the highway, in an open field.

The air-bag ballooned into Luigi, saving his head from crashing through the windshield onto the hood. He was groggy. The shock of the smash left him seeing stars. He reached up and wiped blood from his mouth. The rest of him, though, emerged miraculously intact.

Luigi shook his head and fragments of glass spit around him like rain. "Marco?" he called. "Francesco, Stefano?"

There was no response. Luigi turned his head to find his friends as blood dripped from his mouth onto his Hugo Boss shirt.

Luigi shrieked. A metal fence post had speared the front right windshield, straight into Stefano's chest and then through Marco's. Francesco, like Luigi, was miraculously unhurt. He was crouching like a spy behind the driver's seat.

Beside Francesco, Marco sat still, his eyes open. But the metal post had driven straight through his heart and in a mere eleven seconds, he had bled to death on the rich leather seats of the totaled car.

Luigi's brother, speared first, was still squirming. He was stuck like a kebob. Groaning in pain, his breaths came wheezing out loud.

It was clear to Luigi that his brother was on the verge of death. He shook the bits of glass from his smashed window and pulled himself up and out. He jumped onto the car's dented roof and began to tug on the metal post with what felt like superhuman strength. Stefano's excruciating screams punctured the air and Luigi fell back in panic onto the grassy field.

Had the pole hit Stefano's heart or even his aorta, he would have died instantly. But having missed his organs, the pole had left the man alive.

Drivers passing the wreck stabbed their cell phones for help and two ambulances staffed by doctors and medics capable of Advanced Life Support arrived within minutes. Police secured the scene before ambulances, emblazoned with an orange reflective stripe, bumped along the grass toward the car.

Extricating the passengers was a challenge. Unlike Luigi, the doctors were well aware that a penetrating object, whether a stick, knife or pole, should always be left in place outside of the operating room. Removing it would put the victim at risk of blood streaming out of torn blood vessels inside the wound. The medics waited twenty minutes for fire services to arrive with tools strong enough to cut through the Alfa Romeo. Onlookers watched in amazement as the car popped opened like a tin can and two skewered bodies were gingerly maneuvered out.

The eight-foot metal pole emerged from Stefano's chest wall, having fractured two ribs, narrowly missing a lung, piercing his diaphragm in a downward path, and slashing his liver and gallbladder. Although there were just a few drops of blood escaping the wound, he was hemorrhaging fast into his abdominal cavity and chest. He drifted in and out of consciousness as the rapid infusion of saline through two large intravenous lines worked to keep him alive. His blood pressure hovered dangerously low while his heart raced in an effort to maintain perfusion of his organs.

It was impossible to lay the skewered Stefano down as long as a dead Marco was attached to one end of the spear.

The physician took over. He ordered that the pole be sliced in two, freeing Stefano of Marco's dead weight. Marco was zipped inside a body bag while Stefano was transported like big game from a hunting expedition into the ambulance. The back doors remained partly open to accommodate the long pole. In a seated position, Stefano made the trip to the hospital. He barely registered the sound of the siren wailing into the night.

In the emergency room, the surgeons cut the fence post at each end, leaving a two-foot piece embedded in Stefano. His blood pressure took a nosedive as medical staff pumped unit after unit of blood, platelets and plasma into his system. He was rushed to the operating table but the trauma surgeons were well aware that removing the post prematurely would kill their patient.

In less than one minute, the drug ketamine anesthetized Stefano and he plunged into dreamless sleep. His blood volume was so low that the anesthetist could not find a large central line in his neck or below the clavicles through which blood could be infused faster than through a vein in his arm. The surgeon explored the wound by cutting around the pole. Then he oh-so-carefully performed a partial hepatectomy, removing the ragged lobe of liver as well as the gallbladder, reducing the open rib fractures, repairing the lacerated diaphragm, and leaving a chest tube in place.

Finally, after attaching sterilized industrial clamps to the post, the doctor and his assistants counted one-two-three, and pulled the weapon from Stefano's body. With the post removed and his wound finally closed, Stefano could now enjoy the feeling of lying down again. He was wheeled into the intensive care unit where he remained for the next twenty days, battling infections and transient renal failure.

Months later, despite some chest pain, Stefano returned to most of his daily activities. He did, however, suffer a permanent defect in the right side of his chest due to the absence of his seventh and eighth ribs. Wearing a bathing suit at the beach was not pretty. He could tattoo some awesome creature over the scar, but he'd have to find the right design first. It was a good idea, though, because he couldn't stand the probing questions that made him relive that terror-filled night.

Soon, Stefano was back at school, studying to be an architect. But in his spare time, he made what he considered to be a significant shift in his favorite pastime: video gaming. He transitioned from *Grand Theft Auto* to *Call of Duty*.

EYE SPY

17

Jhatinder was born in Eluru, Andhra Pradesh along the Bay of Bengal on the eastern coast of India. The city lay quietly on the border of the Kolleru Lake and had a population of less than 200,000. But small as it was, Eluru was famous in the region for carpet making, tanning and textile manufacturing.

Jhatinder lived a comfortable middle-class life with his father, a civil servant, his mother, a housewife, and his three younger sisters. But Jhat, as he was known to his friends, hid a secret. He was only fourteen when he started hearing voices. At night, lying in bed, he heard the growling voice of a man tell him to chew his toenails.

At first, Jhat thought the voices were just dreams taking over his mind as he was sinking into sleep. But when he sat up, and turned on the light, he still heard them. The voices even started bickering. One instructed him to pull out his hair while the other suggested he punch himself in the groin.

Jhat tried to silence the voices but they fought him awake every night. They emanated from the flickering shadows cast on the walls of his bedroom from the streetlight outside his window.

Soon, the charming boy his family knew so well began to morph into a moody teen. By the time he graduated high school, he was spending all of his time either eating or locked in his bedroom, doing who knows what. Jhat's parents tried to chalk his behavior up to typical teen stuff. But they noticed that his friends were not so isolated, and when they questioned Jhat, he just shrugged and walked away.

When the savage voices in Jhat's head told him to stay silent, he obeyed. What Jhat didn't know was that his perception of reality was being threatened. When the voices told him not to brush his teeth, he did not, and his breath became unbearable for those around him. When instructed to relieve himself in the kitchen sink, he complied to the horror of his family.

After months of inexplicable behavior, such as collecting his nasal secretions in a giant snot ball on his desk, his parents, ashamed and helpless, sought psychiatric help for their only son. Because Jhat refused to leave the house, the psychiatrist knocked on his bedroom door. Jhat stood facing a balding man in a creased gray suit. The doctor took a seat on the floor, opposite him. He surely had no idea that Jhat was, just then, fighting instructions to shove the man's face into the snot ball.

"Jhatinder, do you know why your parents summoned me?" Dr. Bhatia asked in a kind voice. Approaching sixty years old, he had spent his career caring for schizophrenic patients. Jhatinder blinked, as instructed, every three seconds.

"I am here because your parents are concerned about you, Jhatinder," the doctor explained. "They are worried that you are sick and they have asked me to help you." Again, Jhatinder blinked. I might as well be talking to a fish, the doctor thought. He would have to make a show of it for at least ten minutes, though, because Jhatinder's parents were watching, wringing their hands in the open doorway.

The voices instructed Jhat to stay silent.

Dr. Bhatia handed Jhatinder's parents some papers to sign, and within seconds, their son was certified incompetent and a danger to himself and others. Then two bulky workers dressed in white uniforms appeared. They picked Jhat off the floor and carried him to a waiting truck that drove him to the Eluru Government District Hospital.

Diagnosed with paranoid schizophrenia, Jhat began taking antipsychotic medication. After a few weeks, the voices began to quiet although he could still hear them if he concentrated hard enough. Reality came into sharper focus but it was still hazy when Jhat was discharged to the care of his relieved but anxious parents. The hospital staff needed to make room for new patients on the ward.

"Do not forget," the doctor told them before Jhat left, "you must make sure he takes his pills every day or he could easily relapse."

The first month at home ran smoothly. Jhatinder's sisters

were recruited to monitor the behavior and hygiene of their older brother. The medication made the voices tolerable, although Jhatinder still had to live with them.

In his head, Jhatinder found himself constantly on guard in battle. He was living on the precipice of reality and hallucinations. He had erected a type of shield in his mind. But it was getting harder and harder to keep those voices from shredding his sanity. "Mutiny!" they cried late one August night, raising their decibels, and their swords.

The voices wanted revenge for months of imprisonment. They ordered Jhatinder to act and he felt powerless to ignore their commands.

It was after midnight when Jhatinder padded into the kitchen. As instructed, he pulled open the cutlery drawer and drew out a small knife. Then he squatted down, and one by one, he sawed off two toes.

The pain was intense. It shrieked through him, drowning out the voices shouting for him to continue. He abandoned the act. He stood up.

"Take the knife! Plunge it through your thigh!" a voice said. Jhat looked up. It was the fridge. And it was tall. Taller than he was. Stronger.

He pulled a lovely pointy knife out of the drawer and like a good boy, he did what he was told. He plunged the knife through his thigh, watching as it emerged from the back. Less painful than the toes, he thought, smiling. He did not hear himself cry out, but his father did.

Jhatinder's father rushed downstairs, flicked on the lights and screamed at the terrifying sight before him. There sat

Jhatinder, propped against the bloodstained cupboard, the linoleum floor freckled with blood. A steak knife protruded from his son's left leg. Who had committed this crime? The madman must still be in the house!

Fearing a home invasion, Jhat's father ran to the phone and dialed for help. As he relayed the scene, watching his son sit still in a chair, mumbling an incoherent mixture of English and Telugu, it dawned on him that these wounds must be self-inflicted. The chaos was amplified by the shrieks of four women, who, one at a time, followed the scary sounds to the kitchen carnage.

The wailing sirens of the ambulance and police car became louder and louder until help was ringing the bell. Jhatinder's father relayed to the officers the history of his son's bizarre behavior and recent hospitalization while Jhat spoke unintelligibly to various kitchen appliances. Paramedics wrapped the stumps of his toes and left the knife in his thigh in place. The hilt had broken leaving only the blade. They placed Jhat's toes into a bucket of ice.

Firmly secured to the gurney, Jhatinder and his lovely knife made the trip to hospital. The voices seized the opportunity.

"I'm Dr. Perzo," the bespectacled psychiatrist said to Jhatinder in the emergency room. "I work with Dr. Bhatia. You remember Dr. Bhatia. Don't you, Jhatinder?"

The voices told Jhatinder to smile. He smiled.

"We need to treat your illness," Dr. Perzo said. "We can't have you injure yourself." And with that, he turned his back on his patient. It was late. The staff were tired. The patient was quiet.

The doctor ordered an intramuscular injection of ris-peridone, an antipsychotic drug that would calm Jhat's voices and bring him closer to reality. The pharmacy had just closed, though, so Jhatinder would have to wait until the next morning for his meds. He was so quiet, so docile, the nurses agreed. Such an easy psychiatric patient was a downright pleasure.

After loosening Jhatinder's restraints, the orderlies shut and locked the door to his room. They were as tired as the nurses. No one noticed that the knife blade was still hiding in Jhat's thigh. Except the voices, that is.

Jhatinder followed the instructions without blinking. It hurt, but he was strong, he had handled pain before. The blood was another story. It was gushing fast, and he was no doctor. But he was smart. He pulled off a sock and shoved it into the hole. Grinning and satisfied, he lay back on the pillow but shut-eye eluded him.

Four hours later, at 6 a.m., the nurse returned to check on her favorite patient. She looked at him and screamed, prompting her fellow nurses to run from their station into the room.

Staring at them from the head of the bed was an eyeball. It sat on a pillow trailing its nerves and blood vessels like a comet. Next to the eye, grinning with a sock shoved in an empty socket, sat Jhatinder, his only eye blinking.

Self-mutilation comes in many forms, and is always a sign of significant mental turmoil. Though not always psychotic (characterized by visual, auditory or tactile hallucinations as in schizophrenia), and often a cry for help, the more extreme the mutilation, the greater the likelihood that the lights are on but no one is home.

Jhatinder had used the knife forgotten by medical staff to gouge his eyeball from its orbital home. There was no way to fix the damage. Unlike with a liver or kidney, no amount of ice would keep the eye alive.

Dr. Perzo was so amazed at his patient's act that he kept the eye in a jar of formaldehyde high on a shelf in his office and he watched it staring at him as he went about his work.

HANDS OFF

18

For twelve years, Brannan and Carter had been neighbors. They met when their boys were in school carpool together a decade back, and now they worked together in the assembly line at the truck plant.

Pulling into their driveways on a summer morning, the friends were ready to celebrate the end of a dull night shift behind them. Brannan invited his buddy over for a cold beer to start the day.

"Give me a sec to change and I'll be right over. Cathy's out with the kids till lunch," Carter said. From the fridge, Brannan grabbed four bottles by the neck, loaded up the crook of his other arm with bags of chips and headed out to the porch. He set up the old leather chairs, relics of past living rooms, put up his feet and waited.

A few minutes later, Carter appeared and plopped into the chair with a fart-like oomph from 250 pounds of fat. He twisted open a bottle and let the cold reward slide down his gullet, losing only a dribble on his chin.

The air was thick with humidity. Another scorcher was about to hit.

"You gonna sleep today?" Brannan asked. After a night shift, it was hard to decide whether bed was a good idea. Instead of wasting the day, it might make more sense to hit the pillow right after supper.

"Dunno," Carter said, slightly slurred. "Cathy said she wanted to check out some furniture for the backyard. Ugh. Shopping. Maybe I'll tell her I'm too tired." He rolled his eyes.

"We need more beer," Brannan declared. He pulled himself to standing and made his way back to the fridge. Buzzed from guzzling two beers already, he bumped his shoulder on the doorway as he passed.

Returning, Brannan set down four more bottles and sat. His porch was in need of a paint job or a demolition, and the yard was a mess. Six-foot hedges ringed his property on either side. He hadn't clipped them since the beginning of the season and now branches sprouted like dreadlocks, splayed in all directions. The grass was overgrown, and toys, many broken, littered the walkway. Old tires leaned against the house collecting rainwater in their rims.

In the front yard, a few skinny trees drooped from thirst. Sticking out of the house at a forty-five degree angle was a large Canadian flag, listless and faded.

As the beer spread through him, Brannan decided it was

time to clean up. He kicked Carter's chair to wake him.

"Get up, dude. Help me fix this place," he said with a goofy smile.

"Forget it, man," Carter said, shooting up his middle finger. "Work is done for the day."

"Keep that finger up and you'll lose it," Brannan said. "Come on, I need a hand. This yard looks like shit, not that yours is much better." He gestured to his friend's kingdom next door.

"We'll just collect some garbage, trim the hedges and who knows. Hey, let's hold a garage sale and cash in. Cathy and Deborah will love us. They can go shopping with the spoils," Brannan said.

He kicked Carter's chair again. All it took was a little friendly cajoling and he could convince Carter to do just about anything.

"Think about how great our yards will look," Brannan said. "Wouldn't take much. Just a few cans of paint and dumping some useless junk."

"One more beer and I'll think about it," Carter said. "Work and me never seem to see eye to eye."

Thinking about it was enough. Brannan cracked open another beer and handed it as payment to his friend. Then he started to plan the cleanup.

"Gimme a hand," Brannan said, heading toward the tires against the house. He picked up one under each arm, spilling dirty water and mosquito larvae on his work clothes. Where should he put them? He leaned them on the hedges, basically repositioning them a few feet from their home.

Carter trudged over. "Let's load the tires in the van and

dump them on the way to work," he said. Then, pointing to hedges: "What's with the jungle?"

Brannan laughed. "You got any clippers?"

"Lemme check," Carter said. He lurched through the brush into his own yard.

Brannan, feeling woozy, held onto the house brick for support. He downed the rest of his beer and waited. Minutes later, Carter reappeared with a beer in one hand and no clippers in the other.

"Nada," he said, shaking his head.

Looking around, Brannan spotted the rusting hulk of an old lawnmower that had been left out all winter. "Hey," he said, pointing. "Let's just use that."

"How?" Carter asked. "That thing wouldn't spark if you threw a match on it. And anyway, it's for grass, dummy. Not hedges."

Brannan tapped his temple. "Stick with me buddy," he said. "That mower is our electric clipper."

Carter was confused and sleepy. He watched Brannan lift the mover over to the hedge.

"Needs gas," Brannan said. He found a full red container inside the garage. He slipped on the nozzle and fed fuel into the tank.

"Watch this," he said, yanking the cord. Nothing happened. Brannan tried again and again until he was sweating and heaving. The sun pummeled his back. He was about to give up when to his surprise, the motor grunted and sputtered before catching. The mower's blades spun wildly, protected by the circular metal housing.

"Okay, Brains. What now? Lift it over the hedge and cut?" Carter said, chuckling.

"Exactly." Brannan grinned. "All we need to do is remove the handles. Then we lift it and skim it over the top. Trust me, pal. This is brilliant. Easier than clippers. A new invention."

It seemed like a crazy idea, but Carter just shrugged, took a last swig of beer, and joined his friend in unscrewing the handles from the mower's frame. He started to sweat. This was far from fun, and he was exhausted, but Carter was in for the ride.

"Step back while I start her up," Brannan instructed. "I don't want anything flying out the bottom and cutting your throat." He winked at his friend as he pulled the starter.

The blades whirred.

"Ready to go!" Brannan called. "Pick up your end like we're moving a couch and we'll give those hedges the haircut of the year!"

The friends heaved the body of the mower, oblivious to the mere inches their hands sat to the rotating blades. Teetering from the weight and deaf from the whir, they raised the mower above their heads. Then they positioned themselves on either side of the hedge and moved it back and forth as if they were brushing a dog.

The blades were spinning at ten revolutions per second when Carter lost his grip. The pair repositioned their hands to keep the machine aloft, but it fell to the ground, blood spouting fast onto the rusty spots. Thankfully, the mower fell blades down, or else the half dozen fingers already flying through the air would have been chopped into slices like pepperoni on pizza, never to be reunited with their owners.

Cathy was pulling into the driveway when she heard a frightening mix of machine and human screams. She hit the brakes and raced from her car to the yard next door. Within seconds, she found the motor's switch and clicked it off.

Blood spurted from both Brannan's and Carter's hands faster than one person could staunch it. Cathy ran to the kitchen and grabbed dish towels to press against the men's wounds.

Dialing 911 from her cell phone, she tried to adjust to the horrible sight. Lying on the ground, along with the two moaning men, their hands wrapped in bloody towels, were a batch of human fingers. She knew it was her job to collect them and save them safely on ice. Having seen the men's hands, she had made a quick calculation. She was hunting for twelve digits.

The men were whimpering now. Cathy shivered and composed herself. Well, there goes the outdoor furniture, she thought, surveying the bloody scene. She ran to the house, filled a bowl with ice and grabbed plastic bags.

Near the men, she scooped up nine fingers. Peering over the hedge, she hunted, cursing as sirens wailed closer. Where the hell were they? Cathy began separating branches and soon spotted a middle finger and a ring finger, protruding like Halloween candles. Eleven down, one to go, she thought.

The ambulance arrived with two medics on board. They moved more slowly than Cathy expected. Armed with orange medical bags, the unionized workers approached the men who were wiggling like worms on the blood-soaked earth, hugging their limbs close to their bodies.

Cathy explained that she couldn't find the final finger. She handed over her catch and continued her search while the medics set to work bandaging the men's hands. On stretchers, the patients were attached to iv lines and then off the ambulance flew, sirens blazing, to the hospital.

Cathy knew that whatever help she could provide would give both Carter and Brannan a better chance at survival. So she continued to stoop and, hopefully, scoop that last finger.

Twenty minutes later, she spotted the sausage-like shape covered in grass and dirt. She raced to hospital and proudly handed the finger to the casualty nurse.

"The emerg doctor is in with them now," said the nurse, beaming and blonde in her pink uniform. "Our plastic surgeon is on his way. I'll let you know when you can visit. It'll be before we wheel them into the OR."

Sedated with morphine, the men still had alcohol warming their blood vessels. Their hands were bandaged in what looked like red and white boxing gloves.

Replanting fingers takes hours of microsurgery by highly trained hands. Repair involves attaching bones, tendons, muscles, nerves and most importantly, the blood supply, including both arteries and veins.

Success depends on the degree to which the fingers are mangled and the extent of muscle destruction. When it comes to reattachment, there is only a short window of opportunity. Wait longer than six hours to reattach uncooled digits, or twelve hours for cooled ones, and you might be out of luck.

Carter and Brannan were transferred to a major university hospital where a team of forty specialists worked in shifts to repair their hands. After twenty-eight hours, only a few minutes of which were spent determining what belonged to whom, the surgery was complete. Unfortunately, though, Brannan's middle finger became infected and could not be salvaged. No more flipping the bird on that side.

Days later, still drifting in and out of consciousness, Carter began to sense a disturbing wriggling feeling around his hands. When he complained to the medical staff, they nodded, but no one seemed willing to help. After a few days, the wriggling became unbearable. So feigning sleep, he checked the unwound dressing as the nurse prepared to change it in the middle of the night.

Carter fainted. He had seen a sight even more frightening than a fingerless hand. All over his reattached fingers, there were a dozen brown leeches sucking his blood.

What Carter didn't know was that leeches are sometimes used in surgery to boost blood flow. They act like mini-pumps as the blood vessels begin functioning again after severe trauma. Although it seems counterintuitive, the little creatures also reduce congestion and prevent infections. To avoid fainting, screaming, or maybe even heart attacks, doctors prefer not to let patients know that they have leeches sucking on their blood. It's just easier that way.

VLAD THE IMPALER

19

Vlad had four hot pizzas in the back seat and an address plugged into his GPS, but he drove to the hospital instead. He couldn't make it through his evening shift; the pain was too much. The forty-two-year-old delivery man parked his car and, abandoning the pizzas inside, scurried through the emergency entrance. At the triage desk, he could barely sit. His chest, butt and balls were aching.

Vlad waited his turn as the triage nurse assisted an elderly man reeking of urine into the inner sanctum of the emergency department to be looked after by a physician.

"I need help," Vlad told her. The triage nurse motioned toward a plastic chair, and pen in hand, began her fortieth assessment of the night.

"What's the problem, sir?" She sounded bored. She was

annoyed that the smell of urine still stained the air around her station.

"Pain. I have pain all over," Vlad said in his thick Russian accent. "My chest, my ass, my balls, everything hurts."

The nurse rolled her eyes. It was time to transfer to a nice, cozy suburban hospital where the patients suffered from real problems, like heart attacks and strokes.

Vlad pulled up his shirt exposing multiple large swellings around his nipples. Drops of yellowish liquid dripped down his chest. The nurse noted that the area looked inflamed. Vlad claimed that he had similar lesions on his scrotum and multiple draining sinus tracts on his rear end but did not drop his pants to prove it.

"How long have you suffered from diabetes?" asked the nurse, presuming that Vlad had multiple abscesses.

"Nyet," Vlad answered, shaking his head vigorously, the pain pulling him back to his native tongue.

The nurse cocked her head. "Well, how long have you had these then?" she asked, pointing with her pen to his chest to ensure that her fingers stayed far away.

"Two, three days," he told her.

Vlad pulled down his shirt, and the nurse took his vital signs. Heart rate, fine. Blood pressure, also fine. No temperature elevation. No sign of malnourishment.

"Have a seat," she instructed, gesturing to the waiting room.

The nurse wrote "multiple abscesses" on Vlad's chart and handed it to her colleague. Twenty minutes later, Vladimir Gryova heard his name called. It was his turn.

Inside a curtained cubicle, he repeated the routine with a second nurse before he was told the doctor was on his way. Moments later, a tanned man wearing green surgical scrubs appeared, his hair gray at the temples, a stethoscope draped around broad shoulders.

"Dr. Cooke," he said by way of simple introduction. "What brought you in today?"

"My car," Vlad answered. "It's parked in lot out front."

Another comedian, Dr. Cooke thought. Great. "What seems to be the problem today?" he rephrased.

"My balls hurt, and my chest and ass," Vlad explained. "They're sore and it is getting worse. I need some medicine to fix me."

Dr. Cooke, like the charge nurse before him, thought it was about time he found a nice, quiet job in a rural hospital. Semiretired, he could spend his days treating simple ailments. But not today, clearly. The doctor asked Vlad a series of questions to rule out the possibility of infection. The patient had no constitutional symptoms — no fever, sweats, chills fatigue, weight loss.

Next, he examined Vlad, and found that both of the man's breasts were red and swollen, tender to touch. Like abscesses, they were leaking fluid but this liquid was clear, not murky as would be expected with an infection. Vlad's backside sported a half dozen similar bumps. Most shocking, though, was Vald's scrotum, which was swollen to four times its normal size and draining the same liquid. It looked like he had a softball or two in there.

Dr. Cooke squinted and frowned. This was a mysterious

scattering of lesions. The pattern was oddly confined to three distinct regions. The doctor knew of many conditions that cause swellings, but he couldn't think of one that would present in this manner, with this distribution. There was something strange going on here.

The doctor suspected that bacteria had somehow caused the swellings and to make sure it wasn't also growing in Vlad's blood, he ordered blood cultures. In case of infection, the nurse started an IV, and took multiple swabs of all affected regions. The specimens and blood culture bottles were transported by a porter to the microbiology lab. Vlad was started on antibiotics and admitted to the general internal medicine ward.

After three days, nothing had changed. The microbiology cultures from blood and tissue grew nothing. In the meantime, the swellings were as angry as ever and continued to weep down Vlad's chest and legs. But now Vlad's behavior seemed odd. He denied knowing anything about the source of the unusual condition and was vague when questioned, hiding behind his apparent limited command of English.

On day four of Vlad's admission to hospital, his doctor consulted the dermatology service. Dr. Lerner was a wizened skin veteran. Often all it took for him to establish a diagnosis was a simple glance. But being an old-school physician, Dr. Lerner liked to sit and chat with his patients.

"So Mr. Gryova, tell me," he said, looking into Vlad's eyes. "How exactly did these bumps on your skin start?"

As Vlad recounted his story, it became clear to the seasoned doctor that vital information was missing. He asked for permission to perform a biopsy of the lesions. Vlad shrugged and scribbled his signature on a consent form.

Dr. Lerner's eyes weren't what they used to be, so he took off his glasses to focus on extracting the correct amount of tissue from the middle of the lesion. With hands that couldn't help but shake, he injected local anesthetic into one of the swellings. Then, after waiting a few minutes for lidocaine to take effect, he deftly cut off some tissue and deposited it into a small tube filled with preservative. He dabbed the wound with gauze and sewed it shut with a few stitches.

After stowing the tube in the front pocket of his lab coat, the doctor ambled down to the pathology lab in hopes of establishing a diagnosis. Looking through the microscope at his handiwork, Dr. Lerner saw very little. But it was what he did not see that confirmed his suspicions. Despite a healthy sample, there was very little actual tissue. No lesions were identifiable, just non-specific regions of inflammation and cystic areas around fat cells of the skin. Dr. Lerner diagnosed Sclerosing Lipogranulomatosis. In layman's terms, Vlad's skin was reacting to some foreign body that had made its way inside of him. But what that was the doctor couldn't tell.

That evening, Dr. Lerner, who had a hip replaced two years before, limped into Vlad's room. The patient was lying on his hospital bed, his face as flat as his body. Overhead fluorescent bulbs lit the room. The intravenous line hung beside Vlad, vanishing into his arm beneath the covers.

Dr. Lerner asked about Vlad's background, his upbringing in Russia, immigration, family life, hobbies.

"I graduated from medicine before you were born, Mr.

Gryova," he told Vlad, who just stared. "I have forty-eight years of experience treating patients. It's enough to know you're injecting something into your body. I'm just not sure what — yet. We are going to consult psychiatry to discuss this with you."

"Nyet," Vlad said, shaking his head.

"Well, I can't make you see a professional. This isn't a kindergarten class. But I'll tell you this, young man. If you don't explain how this happened, it may get worse and spread throughout your entire body." Dr. Lerner wasn't really worried about this possibility. But the suggestion might be just what he needed to crack his secretive patient. Vlad looked at the ceiling. Minutes passed. Eventually, he looked at Dr. Lerner and squirmed.

"It may have gotten into my skin by mistake," he whispered.

"What may have?" Dr. Lerner prodded.

"Some liquid plastic that I use."

So that was it. Vlad was purposely injecting liquid plastic into his body. The doctor had heard of cases like this one. Vlad might be suffering from a rare factitious disorder, when a patient pretends to have a disease by creating or exaggerating symptoms.

Self-injection is a well-recognized act in patients with factitious disorder. Foreign materials include silicone, needles, rocks, and even feces. The lesions tend to appear in areas that the patient can reach with a needle. Often, women inject their breasts — a much rarer site for men. Women with this condition sometimes request mastectomies in the absence of a family history of early onset breast cancer or proven genetic susceptibility.

Doctors become suspicious of this disorder when the patient exhibits bizarre personality traits and there is no objective cause for the reaction, such as the case report where a man used a gloved hand to cover one arm in poison ivy. He wanted to make absolute sure that the reaction affected only one of his limbs.

Some factitious disorder patients are termed "malingerers." Like Klinger from the television series *M*A*S*H*, they are motivated to feign illness by financial or some other gain. However, most patients are unaware of their motivations.

Münchausen syndrome is a type of factitious disorder where patients conjure up false symptoms in order to bask in medical attention. Rather than actually harming themselves, these patients concoct reasons for hospital investigation, such as spiking their urine with drops of blood.

In another case, a young man presented to Sunnybrook Hospital in Toronto feigning ventricular tachycardia, or VT, a life-threatening cardiac rhythm disorder. When no one was looking, he shook the ECG leads monitoring his heart. The patient knew that the shaking would result in an electrical artifact on the monitor that is difficult to distinguish from true VT. In fact, having tried this trick before, he had already been prescribed a powerful rhythm controlling medication by an electrical expert at another teaching hospital in Toronto.

Luckily, a part-time nurse working a shift in the emergency room recognized the man from a recent stay at another Toronto hospital where his behavior was identified as suspicious. As it happened, the patient had visited dozens of hospitals, using different names. His medical chart arrived a few hours later and some of his previous escapades where he had fooled medical staff were documented. Now, when the staff asked to photograph him to confirm his identity, the young man bolted, as such patients often do.

Now that Dr. Lerner had discovered the cause of Vlad's lesions, he again offered his patient the chance to consult with a psychiatrist. Vlad was quite sure that he didn't want any doctors poking around inside his brain, however. So, the next morning, he traded the hospital gown for his clothes, and against medical advice, he discharged himself, still weeping fluid and liquid plastic.

BARBIE DOLL

20

It had only been two months and already Luanne was fed up with marriage. She honestly didn't know if she could take another night. She needed a way out.

She was working her shift at the grocery store, yet again, watching oj and apples and Bear Paws making that endless glide along the belt before she lifted each item, one by one, and scanned — beep, beep, beep.

"Price check on 3. Price check on 3," Luanne droned into her microphone. How much were green seedless grapes again? And also, what was with the eleven varieties of each and every fruit? Couldn't they just sell one type of apple and make life easy for everyone? Rather than hunting for the grapes some-where in the store guide stowed beneath her register, Luanne just called for help and over rushed Bradley, head fruit and vegetable stock boy. The lineup collectively scowled, rolled eyes and shifted weight from one foot to another.

The owner of the grapes made smacking sounds as her lipsticked mouth worked a wad of gum. "It's 99¢ a pound," she said. "I checked before I bagged them."

Luanne ignored her and her dyed blonde hair and manicured tips. Customers always claimed to know the prices and nine times out of ten, they were selling her a load of crap.

She turned to Bradley. You could bet he'd have the answer. This dude had an uncanny knowledge of the price of produce at a single glance. In fact, Bradley arrived at work an hour earlier than everyone else just to memorize the pricing changes of fruit and vegetables. He was the Trivial Pursuit produce king.

"Organics," Bradley said, deadpan. "They're $4.99 a pound."

Having done his job, he turned and headed back to his home in produce. Luanne smiled. She loved calling Bradley over for price checks. The more often she saw him at work, the more clearly she could picture his lanky body over her as she was lying there beneath her new, nutty husband.

"That's nuts!" the blonde screeched. "Take them away. I don't want them. Probably full of bacteria anyway."

Luanne absently placed the bag of grapes behind her. She was lost in regret. How could she have missed the signs? The courtship had been long. Long enough to see. And yet, it had all started with such promise.

At first she thought she was losing her mind. The new lace bra and matching thong she had bought to surprise Blaine with was nowhere to be found. She remembered snipping off the tickets and tucking them into her lingerie drawer, but they too were gone. It wasn't as if she kept an inventory of her undergarments, but after a while it became obvious that something was amiss. Whenever she purchased new bras, panties or nighties they either vanished or felt strange somehow when she first put them on.

Was it possible that a voyeur had been spying through the window and had gained access to their apartment when they were out? Luanne had read about such nasty business in the pages of tabloids on the racks at checkout. But it was impossible. She and Blaine rented an eighth floor apartment with a bedroom that faced a brick wall. The superintendent had a key. But the hefty Bulgarian woman could never squeeze into Luanne's 34B cup let alone her size four panties.

It took a few weeks for the uneasy seed of realization to grow in Luanne's mind. First she noticed that Blaine took his sweet time in the bathroom before coming to bed. Next, he seemed increasingly disinterested in conventional sex. In bed, he began asking her to do odd things involving an array of toys. At the same time, sex aids and movies with unusual themes appeared around the apartment. Blaine was taking what seemed to be a passive-aggressive approach to meeting his sexual needs and Luanne wasn't biting.

Despite all of these clues, when her husband emerged from the bathroom last night wearing her brand new satin nightgown, Luanne was shocked.

Blaine saw her mouth fall open and retreated in shame back into the bathroom where he locked the door. Seconds later, having regained her composure and feeling disgust and sympathy rise in equal parts in her chest, Luanne knocked. No answer. Okay, well, she wasn't going to beg. Her husband would come out when he was good and ready. Luanne sighed. In bed alone, she pulled the covers to her neck and nodded off. By the time she awoke this morning, Blaine was gone.

A driver for the gas company, he spent his days loading and delivering propane tanks. Blaine thanked the stars that he had worked for the company since he graduated form high school. Now, he had a job for life. It was this measure of stability that had attracted Luanne in the first place.

These days, that stability she had always craved was showing cracks. Luanne, a good girl, a God-fearing Southern Baptist, thank you very much, now realized she was married to a lace panties wearing, chocolate sex toy eating, latex movie watching freak. Now she'd never have her two kids and white picket fence, she thought miserably, as she scanned and bagged, scanned and bagged.

What was she going to do? Return to her parents who had warned her that, at nineteen, she was far too young to elope?

Luanne dreaded the end of her twelve-hour shift. At 7 p.m., she changed into her T-shirt and jeans and lingered in the coffee room. Then she walked to her apartment block, ten minutes away. At the rate she was going, it took her twenty. By the time she reached the front door of the aged building, she had smoked three cigarettes down to the filter.

The elevator creaked its way up. Luanne got out on seven because the elevator door on her floor was still busted. She took the last flight by stairs. The hallway was dim and dingy.

Luanne stuck her key in the lock and shook the door open with nervous hands. The apartment was quiet.

"Blaine?" she called. No answer. She sighed. "Blaine, I'm home." Silence.

Maybe he was so full of shame that this was it, Luanne thought. Maybe he was never coming back and would face her next in divorce court.

She put away the grocery items she had lugged home from work: three cans of baked beans, a jar of low fat mayonnaise, four tins of tuna in water, a jug of pulpy orange juice, a carton of Matinée Extra Mild, a second of Player's Light and, as a special treat, two Japanese apple pears. Then she lit another cigarette, fell into the living couch and clicked on the TV.

She spent the next half hour channel surfing, letting banal talk show banter bounce off her brain. But she was preoccupied. Visions of her husband in various forms of lingerie danced before her. So eventually, she clicked it off and headed to the bedroom. She would figure this out. She just wasn't sure how or when. Maybe tomorrow would bring answers.

For a second, Luanne thought he was sleeping on the bed, but when she moved closer, she saw that her husband's head was shiny. She bent down and saw that over his features was a second skin — a clear plastic bag. She briefly considered that someone crazed had murdered Blaine. Lying diagonally across the comforter face up, his eyes were fixed on the stucco ceiling. His mouth hung open like a thirsty dog. Luanne shrieked and fled the apartment. Racing down the stairs, she fumbled with her cell phone and called her mother.

The police arrived, followed soon after by the county

coroner, Dr. Dung Nguyen. Yellow police tape sealed the apartment. Two bald cops guarded its entrance. The death was another misadventure but how and why had it occurred?

The coroner had seen many similar cases in her career. Blaine looked stylish in a magenta bra stuffed with toilet paper, and over it, a purple nightgown with flowered straps. Luanne recognized the set instantly. She had worn it on her wedding night. On her husband's head was a clear plastic bag connected by a rubber tube to a barbecue gas tank. Beside the tank sat a tube of lubricant and a collection of naked Barbie dolls. The dolls, manufactured without evidence of genitalia, had pubic hair and nipples applied with crude nail polish strokes.

It turned out that Blaine, his corpse already beset by rigor mortis by the time his wife had discovered it, had died when Luanne was still at the store. After finishing work at noon, he had been excited when he entered the empty apartment and could take advantage of the opportunity to play alone. And what a party it had been. Postmortem X-rays identified yet another Barbie doll, this one in Blaine's rectum, sheathed in a balloon. Dr. Nguyen elected not to verify the presence of a paint job on that one.

The cause of death was ruled accidental. Blaine had asphyxiated after inhaling propane, resulting in an autoerotic death. There were variations on this theme, and Dr. Nguyen had seen too many to count. The victim engages in auto-erotic practices to heighten sexual arousal. Those who enjoy the feeling of reduced oxygen in the lungs to boost sexual gratification are called gaspers. Death results when a gasper accidentally goes too far and suffocates. In this case, when Blaine fell unconscious with pleasure, he had no way to shut off the gas or remove the bag.

Against her parents' better judgment, Luanne remarried. But this time, she Googled as many sexual paraphilias as she could find before she committed to till death do us part. Marriage was going to be more fun the second time around.

A CUT ABOVE

21

The foreskin — that small slice of flesh that Jews do away with in the first few days of a boy's life — is classified as being "functionally redundant." The question is: does it serve a purpose?

Besides protecting what is arguably a man's most sacred head from harsh uv rays during nude sunbathing, the foreskin does nothing for the body. And yet, we humans aren't alone. Almost all mammals have one — including the twenty-year-old man who presented to the emergency department of a small hospital in a sleepy town in the southern United States.

Bent over in agony, he shuffled to the front desk clutching his groin with both hands as if he had just been hoofed by a horse. His eyes were bloodshot. His tear-stained face was contorted. Through his teeth, he groaned for help.

Becky, the triage nurse with decades of big city experience

behind her, pegged his case as appendicitis or perhaps a kidney stone, and yet the man did seem a bit young. Supporting him under her arm, she escorted the patient to a gurney parked against the wall of the triage area. He struggled onto the stretcher.

"What seems to be the matter?" Becky asked in her light English accent.

In answer, Peter rolled into a fetal ball, facing her. That's when the nurse saw his blood-stained hands. There was also a wet splotch on the crotch of his jeans.

"You must tell me what happened," Becky insisted. Alarmed, she checked his vital signs. This was no burst appendix. Clearly, this man had been either shot or stabbed. Although gang violence was still mainly an urban problem, even small towns were becoming plagued by drug wars.

When she worked in a large city hospital, Becky had seen the aftermath of dozens of shootings and stabbings. She knew that this man's femoral arteries were intact; an injury to the large arteries of the legs could cause a person to drop dead from blood loss within a single minute. Judging by the softball-sized bloodstain, Becky assessed that, thankfully, Peter was in no danger of exsanguinating. There just wasn't enough blood.

With a porter's help, Becky directed the oversized gurney wheels to a cubicle in the acute care area. Peter stayed silent. His breaths came out fast and his heart rate jumped, but his blood pressure remained normal.

Becky looked at the man who still hadn't uttered a word. "Suit yourself," she said, as she plunged a plastic intravenous catheter into a vein in Peter's arm. Cool saline flushed through the tube and mingled with his warm blood. She cracked open the IV and started a liter saline bolus, just in case.

"Take off your clothes and I'll send in the doctor," Becky said. "You're going to have to tell someone what happened to you, young man." She turned and left.

Inside the cubicle, Peter moaned as he inched down his pants. He kept his blood-soaked shirt on, stretching it down to hide his groin.

Dr. Cohen, urgently summoned by the nurse, brushed aside the curtains and rushed to Peter. Becky followed. Believing on sight that the patient had been shot or stabbed in a drug deal gone sour, he asked the nurse to inform security. Caution was key in moments such as these.

The doctor introduced himself and without asking a question, lifted the young man's hands with his own gloved ones, and inspected the wound. The blood seemed to be trickling from the end of poor Peter's penis. A careful check confirmed that his testicles as well as the remainder of his groin were unscathed. The bits of dried blood were harmless. Bending over, Dr. Cohen saw that a jagged tear encircling the member was oozing dark blood. And yet, the rest of the penis appeared intact.

To stem the bleeding, the doctor wrapped the wound with sterile gauze. Reassured that the laceration was, while obviously painful, neither deep nor life threatening, Dr. Cohen tried to figure out how such a strange, selective injury had occurred. With twinkling eyes, he asked the obvious question: "What did you do?"

Peter stayed silent.

"Well?" the doctor asked. Still, nothing. "Listen," he continued. "I hate to do this. But you have to understand the predicament I'm in here. This injury looks suspicious, possibly the result of a violent encounter, maybe even illegal activity. And it's my job to get to the bottom of it. Just in case there is something I need to report to police."

That was it. The thought of a line of cops marching into the room to inspect the damage was just too much. As painful as it was to relive what had happened, Peter would talk. He'd talk now.

Peter looked into the doctor's eyes, and in a shaky voice, he began. "Well, Doc. I was surfing the Net, you know, and I saw this really interesting site. It was called Freedom from Foreskin."

The doctor nodded, urging him on.

"I'd been, you know, smoking some weed, just for fun, and I, well, I've always wanted to be circumcised. I'm not sure why my parents never had me circumcised. I mean pretty much all my friends were. So it's kinda weird, you know?"

"Go on," Dr. Cohen said, seeing just where this story was headed. Peter detailed the self-surgery: How he had followed the step-by-step instructions on the screen, and protected his penis from a possible errant nick by slicing the top off a water bottle and poking the head of his penis through. Then, he'd sprayed the head with topical anesthetic purchased at the pharmacy, and with his mother's tweezers he had grasped his panicked foreskin through the hole.

"I waited fifteen minutes to make sure I wouldn't feel a thing, just like the website said," Peter told the doctor.

Dr. Cohen's eyes grew wide. He was biting down on his molars, forcing his face to look calm.

"That's when I grabbed the little scissors my mother keeps in her bathroom drawer, and well, I snipped."

It was the doctor's turn to remain silent.

"It didn't go too badly at the start," Peter said. "It stung a bit, which was odd since the website said it would be painless. But the problem was I couldn't stop the damn bleeding. I kept rubbing it. Maybe I rubbed off the anesthetic, I don't know. And then what do you know, I got an erection, from all the rubbing I guess, and it started to bleed more. It started to sting something awful. I couldn't stand it. My dick was killing me. The pain was so bad I drove myself here."

Dr. Cohen's molars were grinding together, hard. They were keeping his face a mask so he wouldn't let the laughter, which was trapped in his throat, fizz into the room. He nodded, shaking, and left, only to return ten minutes later, composed, and carrying a needle.

"Okay, young man," he said. "You've been through worse."

Carefully, the doctor grasped Peter's penis, and jabbed its base, letting the anesthetic liquid find its mark: the nerve carrying all of the sensory information to and from it. Within minutes, Peter's member was numb and finally, the agony dissolved.

Later that evening, the town's general surgeon repaired Peter's amateur hatchet job. After just ten minutes, his circumcision was finally complete. On the way out of the hospital, Peter grabbed a fistful of complimentary gauze pads. Just in case.

SPLIT SECOND

22

Pieces of a body were freshly strewn along the railroad tracks of a small Spanish town. The train that had just run over a man remained parked on the tracks almost a mile from the scene, still dripping blood from its engine.

Carlos, chief medical examiner for the municipality, walked toward the gruesome scene. As he did, his trained eye stopped at each body part, examining what was left of the well-dressed corpse. Carlos finally arrived at the torso. What a waste of an Armani suit, he thought.

With a gloved hand, he pinched the dead man's bloody wallet from the blazer pocket and flipped through its contents. Everything seemed to be intact: driver's license, Visa gold card, American Express, $1,800 in cash. An HSBC identification card with the man's photo revealed he was a banker. Carlos did the math: He was forty-eight.

Every day, around the world, people are killing themselves, Carlos thought. They jump off bridges, tie nooses around necks, shoot drugs, drink poison, pull triggers, dive into deep, freezing water. Often, there seems to be no logic to how it's done. But suicide, he knew, is usually an act of convenience and opportunity fueled by depression or the influence of drugs and alcohol. And there is no getting around the fact that cities bordering bodies of water are home to more drownings, and countries with lax gun laws more likely have gunshot wounds as a leading cause of their citizens' deaths.

When it came to suicide, Carlos knew even more. He was aware that the three countries with the highest reported suicide rates are Belarus, South Korea and Lithuania. In the United States, suicide is the eighth leading cause of death in males and nineteenth in females. In young people, between the ages of fifteen to twenty-four, it is the third leading cause (behind accidents and homicide), but the rates are highest in those aged thirty-five to forty-nine.

But as common as suicides may be, Carlos was careful not to jump to conclusions. The first question was: Was this an accident, homicide or suicide? And other questions followed: Were the injuries to the corpse inflicted at another location? Was it dragged here? Was the scene staged to look like a suicide to deflect blame? For experienced forensic investigators like Carlos, these types of questions can fly around for a long time until they are finally answered.

After taping off the scene and directing the police photographer to shoot the various body parts, Carlos approached the shaken engineer, who was sitting cross-legged in the field with his head in his hands.

"Hey, buddy," Carlos said.

The engineer, whose name was Jose Luis Maldanado, looked up with hollow eyes. "There was no stopping," he said.

Jose Luis understood that trains hit people all the time. He had one friend, Armando, who had hit three in his career. Poor Armando. He felt forced to retire. The nightmares — reliving those final moments of braking, the train refusing to stop — kept haunting his dreams. He was a grandfather, for God's sake.

But Jose Luis hadn't seen this coming.

"Just take me through it, step-by-step, Mr. Maldanado," Carlos said. His pen was poised on his notepad, but he also had his tape recorder on, peeping out of his breast pocket. There was no telling where this one would go.

"I was rounding a curve in the tracks so I'd slowed to fifty miles per hour," Jose Luis said. "And there he was, lying straight across."

He explained how he had activated the brake system, knowing full well that he needed a mile of track to come to a complete stop. He immediately blew the train's horn, all 140 decibels of ear-shattering warning.

"It should have scared the daylights outta him, should have made him jump up, but he just turned his head toward the train," the engineer said, shaking his own head now.

"He didn't jump up," Carlos said.

"No. He had the chance to roll off — I was still 300 yards away — but instead, he did something I will never forget."

Carlos scribbled fast, then he flipped a page, and waited.

"He had been lying across both tracks, his head over one side, his legs dangling over the other," Jose Luis recalled. "Then, as the wheels screeched, the man started to move. I thought he was getting up. I thought he was saved. And then, instead, he lay back down again, this time positioning himself longitudinally along the length of one of the two tracks. I've seen dozens of suicides in thirty years on these lines, but I've never seen anyone looking to get split into two equal parts."

Carlos scratched at his pad, shaking his head. Suicide.

"What next?" Carlos asked.

"What could I do? It was clear the guy had chosen this particular site, just around a curve, knowing I would not be able to stop in time. So I did all I could do. I kept the brake on, and turned my head. Many seconds passed. I felt just a soft bump. That's it. The train barely registered the impact. We stopped about half a mile from the body and I called police. Done."

"Jeez," Carlos said. All of the voluntary train deaths he had seen were pure decapitations. There are two pieces of the corpse to identify — head and body and that's it. Accidental train deaths, on the other hand, are messy. The forensic scene is often characterized by severe injuries including multiple fractures and extensive soft tissue trauma, reflecting the victim's attempts to evade being shredded by hundreds of tons of speeding steel.

In this unusual case, the body was literally split down the

middle as the train decelerated on its fatal journey. Shortly after impact, the internal organs spilled out and were dragged hundreds of yards down the tracks as the train slowed. Although the body was dissected, it was hardly a clean and surgical transection. Parts of the man lay everywhere. In the end, only his limbs were anatomically intact.

Not surprisingly, the family decided against an open casket and opted for cremation. At least that way, they would have all of the man in one place.

THE COKE SIDE OF LIFE

23

Nathan Smith was pissed off. He marched out of the gym and down the dimly lit school hallway, punching random metal lockers along the way until his knuckles were oozing blood.

Nathan had the loping gait of a teenager. He was dressed in a white T-shirt a size too big for his skinny frame and red shorts so loose that two of his friends could have joined him in there. The outfit he considered the ultimate in cool was completed by his $300 high-top All-Star basketball sneakers. Nathan was smelly with sweat, and his long hair, damp from an hour of dribbling practice, clung to his head. To make matters worse, he was thirsty.

"Fucking coach," Nathan muttered. "Never fucking satisfied. Always yelling and screaming. I'm sick of this bullshit." He scowled as he snaked through the school's halls, unable to escape the stink of disinfectant sprayed by the night cleaning staff.

For the past three years running, Nathan was proud to boast, he had been the starting center on the JWC Raiders, Class 1 Division Champs. At seventeen, he was now in his senior year and final season. Ask anyone: he was by far the best player on the team.

With hopes of a university basketball scholarship floating within reach, Nathan was a hot commodity in Topeka, Kansas. A few scouts had already expressed interest, traveling the country to watch him dominate in his last home game against the Shelnot High Bombers.

But the moment that first scout came sniffing, something strange happened. Nathan's relationship with Coach Linsky, which had always been solid and respectful, suddenly snapped. Where once, the coach would have patted him on the back for attempting a three-point shot from way downtown, now Nathan found himself the target of ridicule.

"What the hell are you doing out there, Smith?" the coach shouted for all the players to hear.

"What the hell do you think I'm doing? My nails?" Nathan wanted to shout back. But he didn't. The coach was, well, his coach. And even if he was behaving like a championship bastard, the guy deserved his team's respect.

But Nathan was getting pretty sick of the fact that the coach took every opportunity to berate and intimidate him on the court during practice. Was Coach Linsky getting too old for this job? Was he jealous of Nathan's talent? Was he frustrated by his inability to escape the small town he was trapped in?

Coach Linsky, however, saw things differently. He was doing Smith the favor of a lifetime. If scouts were coming to watch his star player, he'd give them something to see.

"The kid's got serious potential," the coach told his wife when he came in the door after a two-hour practice that made his players look like they had just taken showers. "And you can bet your life I'm going to make sure the world sees it."

Unfortunately for Nathan, he was too young and inexperienced to realize that the coach was trying to bring out his best. Feeling deflated after each practice, Nathan now seemed lethargic during games. The harder the coach worked him, the less Nathan seemed to work. He was losing his edge.

Then, during a playoff game against the Bombers, Nathan found himself at his breaking point. That day, Nathan Smith played as if he was the only guy on the team. Sure he was the most talented player, but after watching him shoot and dribble with every possession, the players and the coach were fuming. When the whistle blew, Nathan knew what was coming.

"Bench, Smith!" Coach Linsky shouted.

"No way!" Smith shouted back, kicking off ten minutes of verbal attack.

Standing there, taking it, Nathan stared at his shoes to keep his feet from kicking this asshole in the crotch.

"That's it. I'm done," he finally muttered before striding toward the double doors leading out of the gym.

"Sit your ass down on that bench!" the coach called after him. "Or you're done all right! You'll be off the team for good!"

Nathan kept walking, kicked open the door with all his force, and didn't stop until he reached the vending machines tucked into a small room beside the cafeteria. The echo of the coach's shouts was still following him when he dug into his pocket for quarters.

Nathan was parched. He had given his all, he told himself. But the truth was, dealing drugs for extra cash meant late night delivery runs that were catching up with him. To play hard, he needed more sleep. But to be able to buy goodies — like brand new Nike high-tops, for instance — he needed more than his weekly allowance. And with all these practices, there was no time for a real job. And besides, he wasn't a druggie himself; he only rarely sampled his wares. But the truth was, the blow was hard to resist sometimes.

Nathan slipped six quarters into the slot, listening to them tinkle one at a time as they dropped. Cold cola beckoned him from behind the glass, and he slapped the button to release it. Nothing happened. He pressed again, harder. Again nothing.

His ears red, arms tired, and throat dry, Nathan was about to blow. He had the buck and a half, a freaking gouge if you asked him, and he was getting his drink, damn it! No one and nothing was going to screw him. Not the school, not the coach, and definitely not this machine.

Nathan banged on the glass, first with one fist, then with both before he started kicking like mad with his $150 shoe. When that didn't work, he grabbed his massive adversary's sides and rocked back and forth. It budged. He rocked harder until with a crash, three cans of Coke flew from its mouth onto the floor.

"Now that's more like it!" Nathan said, breaking into a

grin. He picked up a can and popped it open. Pop sprayed like a fountain celebrating his victory. Nathan chugged.

"Cheers, baby," he said to the machine, holding up the open can. He figured he deserved as many free drinks as he could rock out of it. So he grabbed his victim again, swaying, slowly at first. The machine was losing its balance, ready to tip, and Nathan hung on, holding it on a slant. Two more cans rolled onto the floor, followed fast by another six, one of which suddenly spilled its contents onto the floor.

Stepping into the Coke, Nathan's feet flew from under him and he slid backward, losing his grip on the machine. Almost immediately, it fell forward, and crashed on top of him, crushing his chest, fracturing all of his anterior ribs, splitting his sternum.

Unable to expand his broken chest, Nathan suffocated, unaware that he was taking his last breath. Blood vessels popped in his conjunctivae leaving pinpoint hemorrhages called petechiae dotting his eyes. There was soft tissue bleeding throughout his chest consistent with asphyxiation.

A half hour later, after the home team lost its game 76–71, the coach went hunting for Nathan to blame. He found him purple and swollen beneath the machine, lying in a sticky pool of Coke, cans lying innocently around him. Coach Linsky shouted for help.

Nathan's stunned teammates rushed to the scene. On three, they heaved the metal coffin off their fallen comrade, but they were too late. All they could do was watch as Nathan was carted into the back of the coroner's station wagon.

The autopsy report noted a stash of crack cocaine stuffed in the deceased's sock, but no traces of the drug in his system. As a result, the pathologist concluded there was no relationship between the cocaine and the cause of death.

In the end, Nathan's life came down to the following little-known facts:

- A pop vending machine is typically nearly seven feet tall
- Loaded with cans, it weighs more than 1000 pounds
- Its center of gravity allows it to be rocked until the point at which the equilibrium is passed
- Soda pop vending machine tipping was reviewed in a 1992 study. Sixty-four injuries were documented, of which sixty-three involved young men. Fifteen deaths were reported in this study as well as thirteen cases of severe trauma.

And finally, there is more than one type of coke that can kill a man.

MAN'S BEST FRIEND

24

Hunting was Tom's favorite pastime. Having grown up in rural Minnesota, he had fond memories of weekend trips with his dad and two younger brothers that ended with fabulous photos of the men holding dozens of dead animals in the air. On Sundays at dusk, the three boys would squish together on the two-hour ride home inside the paneled station wagon, sharing space with a load of bloodied bird carcasses in the trunk. Like hockey games on the frozen pond, the family's hunting trips carried on into manhood.

Tom's family had lived under the central flyway, a major North American duck migration route, for generations. One of four main paths, the flyway traversed the Great Plains from Canada to the Gulf of Mexico. As a result, Tom was comfortable firing at all types of animals.

His bungalow walls boasted the prizes of his twelve-gauge shotgun. In room after room, dozens of mounted heads stared at each other in frozen wonder. Although there were a few deer and moose, Tom tended to kill Minnesota fowl, which included ducks, geese, mourning doves and pheasants. His bird of choice was the mallard duck with its bright green head and purple speculum. He puffed with pride stringing together a dozen drakes at the neck then slinging his catch over his shoulder at the day's end.

Duck hunting was on the decline in Minnesota, and the number of hunters was dropping year by year until there were only about 60,000 left. Big-game hunters, on the other hand, were flourishing as tales of enormous black bears, elks with huge racks and white-tailed deer attracted those hoping for a trophy from all over the continent. Tom couldn't give a crap, though. He could have been the only duck hunter in the entire state and he'd be happy.

"I'm clocking out!" Tom yelled at the end of a long day on the job. He had worked the night shift in shipping and receiving at the purchasing department of Osterhose Dairy Works for the past fifteen years. The job was as dull as dishwater but health benefits kept him hooked. A decade from now, he saw himself retired, spending his days hunting instead of boxing, taping and mailing.

"Hunting this weekend?" asked Kevin, his coworker. It was a rhetorical question.

"Yep. Truck's already loaded," Tom said. "I've been waiting all week. Going home to round up the dogs and my brothers and in a couple of hours, I'm free as a bird." He gave Kevin a wink.

Anyone who hunts ducks has dogs. And the best duck hunting dogs are retrievers, the most popular breed in the world, because they are not only loyal companions but also seem to enjoy the sport. Tom's four-year-old butterscotch Lab retriever, Ollie, had webbed feet that made him ideal for the cold, wet duck hunting environment. Tom cheered the dog on as he barreled into the water and almost instantly recovered dead or injured birds. Ollie truly was Tom's best friend.

Tom swung his truck around the bend to his brothers' house, headlights shooting through the rural dark. Tim and Ted still lived at home. There was no need to honk; his brothers were sitting on the porch waiting. They nodded a tired hello at Tom then spent the hour-long drive on unpaved two-lane roads alternating between mumbling and sleeping. Tom resorted to talking to Ollie, who hung on his every word.

At dawn, the truck arrived at the perimeter of Iron Lake. Tom parked in a field and the three men, trailed by their dogs, lumbered out.

It was late autumn. The rising sun splashed orange light on the crop. Tom leaned against the cab of his Ford F-150, an unlit cigarette mashed between his lips. He enjoyed the early morning silence before the shotgun made it jump to life. Ollie paced around the truck, yelping with the other dogs as Tom and his brothers collected their gear. Tired as they were, they were ready to kill as many birds as the law would allow. Hunting was a blast. Getting up at four in the morning, not so much. But now that the boys were all here, Tom was spiked with adrenaline. He had been awake since yesterday afternoon.

"Ready boys?" yelled Ted. "Let's take Iron Lake!"

"Lemme check my gun again," Tom said. He used a Remington 870 Wingmaster pump-action shotgun, along with the millions of other hunters who had discovered the model since it hit the market back in 1950. Tom was proud of the fact that his gun held the record for best-selling shotgun in the history of the world. Ever careful, Tom lifted his firearm from the cab of his truck with the hands of a new father and slung that baby over his shoulder.

Blued steel with a satin walnut stock, the Remington glistened in the early light. Its three shell internal tube magazine was empty, as Tom never loaded the gun until he was ready to launch. Sporting neoprene hip waders with lug soles, Tom dropped in the shells as Ollie pranced around awaiting his master's go.

Iron Lake was a silent ten-minute walk from the field where the truck was parked.

"Tom! Your turn on the decoys!" yelled Tim, the middle brother.

No one liked to set the decoys, but they were perhaps the most important of all of the hunting equipment. Wading into the mucky water so early in the day was murder. But it was Tom's turn. So he collected the bag of molded plastic ducks, laid his rifle on the bank and headed into Iron Lake, leaving Ollie whining onshore. Tom pulled a weighted decoy from his bag and threw it. He planned on spreading the decoys thirty yards apart. Just as he was about to grab a second from the bag, Tom heard a shot ring out, and he plopped like a stone into the still water.

Ted jumped off the cooler and raced into the lake. He grabbed his brother by the scruff of the neck and dragged him to shore. There was a bloody hole in Tom's forehead.

Hunting injuries, as former United States Vice President Dick Cheney will attest, are all too common. In North America alone, about a thousand hunters per year are accidentally shot and about one hundred of those shots are fatal. But this case was unusual. Here, the murderer whined and jumped on his victim, licking his face.

Tom had left the loaded firearm on the bank of the lake pointing toward the water. In a cruel and crazy twist of fate, the dog had, in his excitement to hunt, stepped on the trigger of his master's Remington. The gun's munition flew forth, sinking steel birdshot and a plastic wad into Tom's brain and instantly killing him.

During the investigation that followed, the police found nothing suspicious. Other than perhaps a lighter than expected trigger pull, the gun had no mechanical deficiencies. It worked fine. The problem is that in the end, it worked a little too fine.

CHICKEN LITTLE

25

Oblivious to the chicken's journey from cage to slaughterhouse, Ernest bit into the succulent meat slathered in hot barbecue sauce. His shirt was already stained orange. Four pints into the evening, he barely had time to chew before swallowing his huge plate full of fast food.

There was nothing dainty about Ernest. Or his feeding habits. With 250 pounds on his six-foot frame, he was, let's say, not much of a salad and lentil kind of guy.

Ripping meat from bone, Ernest suddenly choked as a pain stabbed his upper chest in the midst of his drunken feast. Coughing, he spit the mashed food onto a paper napkin then gulped the dregs of his beer.

He pounded his chest, trying to force a burp. The pain subsided but he could still feel a burn. To douse it, Ernest reached for his glass of lukewarm table water. He coughed again, chased the water with another glass of beer, burped, then repeated the cycle a few more times.

"You okay, man?" asked his buddy, Dylan.

"Swallowed funny," Ernest rasped. "Feels like something's stuck in my throat."

Ernest threw some bills on the table, mumbled to Dylan that he had to get up early the next morning and left the bar. He walked the two blocks to his basement apartment, with the burn in his chest zinging each time he took a breath. Drunk and uncomfortable, he collapsed, fully clothed, on his unmade bed. Moments later, he was snoring, and drooling onto the sheets.

Three hours later, the need to pee woke him up. Ernest dragged himself to the bathroom but not before veering into the wall. Targeting the toilet, he managed to mostly hit the waiting water. But he still felt a nagging ache in his chest. He stumbled back to bed and awoke the following day just after noon.

As usual, Ernest rolled out of bed with a raging hangover, replete with a mouth that tasted like cotton, so he padded to the kitchen and tipped a carton of iced tea straight down his gullet. He popped a couple of aspirin tablets to clear his headache, then sat on the toilet, dumped his load, and stood up.

Ernest was surprised to see a black tarry trail in the water. What had he eaten? Obviously something that had turned bad. He flushed and washed his hands. Then, feeling lightheaded, he flopped back onto his mattress and snoozed. After finishing the night shift, Ernest had nowhere to spend his afternoons but the bar.

As days became weeks, Ernest continued to feel low so he called his family doctor. She said the black poop was likely the result of an ulcer, and after prescribing an antacid for the ache, she arranged blood tests. Then came the bad news: no more alcohol, no more drugs. Ernest figured he could live without crack cocaine, but beer? Well, that was a problem.

Later that day, a voice called out to Ernest from his answering machine. It was the doctor.

"I need to talk to you about your blood tests. Come in tomorrow — anytime," she said. Ernest wasn't surprised. His poop was still coming out like tar and he was more tired than usual.

Sitting in the waiting room, Ernest felt fear itching inside of him. The chair was too small for his frame and he felt glued to the vinyl. Each time he shifted, it was as if more of him became stuck. He wondered if anyone's ass had ever been scraped like gum off one of these waiting room chairs.

"Ernest Gliadin," the secretary called, and Ernest peeled himself up and followed the woman into the doctor's office. The doctor stood and greeted Ernest with a worried smile.

"I'll get right to the point, Ernest. Your blood count is low," she said.

Ernest stayed silent and Dr. Ross continued.

"We measure something called hemoglobin as part of your blood tests. When people bleed or don't manufacture enough blood cells, it's reflected in the hemoglobin count. The normal number is around 140 or 150 and yours is 100. And with your history of melena — the tarry poop you reported — it confirms that you are indeed bleeding."

CHICKEN LITTLE

The doctor went on to say that she suspected the presence of an ulcer. She explained that people who drink too much alcohol are more prone to them. Ernest would need to be scoped by a gastroenterologist the next day.

"Can't we just stick with meds, Doc?" Ernest liked meds. In fact, he loved them. They were drugs, and what on God's given earth was better than drugs? Nothing. And let's face it, the last thing he wanted was someone shoving a tube down his throat.

"I'm feeling better," he told the doctor, trying to convince both her and himself. "Really. I think the pills are helping."

"I'm worried about you, Ernest," the doctor soothed. "A hemoglobin of 100 is not subtle. If we don't catch the source of this, your health can decline."

She leaned over the table and looked deep into Ernest's eyes. "Ernest, this is not really a negotiation," she said. "This is what you need, and I want you to understand that if you don't follow my advice, there is a chance you could die."

Oh please. Talk about melodramatic, Ernest thought. What am I, cast in an after-school special? She was sweet, though, with her motherly concern. It made Ernest feel loved.

He grinned. "I'll think about it, Doc," he told her, intending not to bother. "Those drugs you gave me are working, I can feel it. And if the pain gets worse, I'll come right back. Promise." He crossed his heart with his finger.

"Call me right away if you change your mind, okay?" the doctor said.

Ernest stood up and left, shaking his head.

Truth was, though, Ernest wasn't feeling better. With each

day, his limbs felt looser, and he kept blackening the toilet water. Just one week after he left the doctor's office, he could not even stand. From bed, he reached for the phone and dialed 911.

Ernest was barely conscious when the super let the medics into his apartment.

"BP 70 by palpation. Heart rate 120," the medic called.

Ernest heard the words like a fading echo. He could hardly feel the plastic catheter enter his vein. Only after a second IV line was inserted and a liter and a half of Ringer's lactate infused into his blood did he perk up enough to discover he was in the back of a bleating ambulance speeding to the hospital.

In triage, it was difficult to keep Ernest's blood pressure steady. He lay there, pale, sweaty and unconscious. The surgeon, Dr. Chu, knew he had little time to get inside Ernest's body and figure out what was wrong.

He prepared to perform a laparotomy, where, through a midline vertical incision in the abdominal wall, he would access Ernest's organs. Aware that Ernest might not survive even the short elevator ride up to the surgical suite, Dr. Chu made sure his patient was anesthetized in the emergency room where the operation would take place.

With Ernest's body gaping on the table, the surgeon found blood spouting from the upper end of his patient's esophagus. Dr. Chu cursed aloud as he tried to stem the flow. It was impossible to find the source of the problem with so much brisk blood. Sponge after sponge was soaked red. In an effort to normalize Ernest's disrupted physiology, the team infused him with unit upon unit of packed red blood cells, platelets and freshly frozen plasma.

When Ernest's heart stopped, the team tried desperately to resuscitate him. But the massive blood loss was too much for the young patient's body. Dr. Chu, quite sure that this had been a readily reversible problem, felt sick himself. He could never quite believe it when his top-notch surgical skills failed.

In life, the source of Ernest's bleeding had been impossible to locate. In death, however, it was easy. The autopsy knife had greater leeway than the surgical scalpel for if it slipped, or cut too deeply, there was no risk to the patient.

Within mere minutes, the pathologist was holding a small chicken leg bone in the air. It had eroded its way through Ernest's upper esophagus, leaving a hole and broken blood vessels. Evidence of chronic inflammatory changes and enlarged lymph nodes indicated that the bone had been hanging out inside Ernest for some time.

While most people think that chicken bones are fatal only when they cause choking, here, it killed Ernest by slowly perforating his esophagus until it caused massive gastrointestinal bleeding.

In fact, pointy foreign bodies, like toothpicks, fish, and chicken bones, are more likely to perforate the esophagus than lower parts of the gastrointestinal tract such as the stomach or intestines. The sharp item, if it doesn't cause a choking death, usually passes straight through the digestive system on its way to the toilet. But rarely, it gets stuck and wreaks havoc. Resulting abscesses, hemorrhaging and even migration of a bone to other parts of the body, such as the heart or lungs, have all been reported.

These injuries occur most commonly in the presence of alcohol and drug use, poor dental habits, and impaired mental states because people with these problems are less likely to properly chew their food. As a result, a blind starving old demented alcoholic drug addict with missing teeth should probably steer clear of chicken and fish.

KENTUCKY WOMAN

26

Rita was the prisoner of an inherited belief system. According to her parents, the modern world presented too many temptations for both children and adults. So they protected her and her seven siblings from the vices of the outside world as if they were all living in a mini North Korea rather than small town Kentucky.

The greatest threat was boys. Rita's parents ensured that their daughter had very little contact with them. They allowed no television or computer in the house. The town's fundamentalist church was Rita's only relationship outside of her family. She had been home-schooled, and was forbidden to step off the family farm unless chaperoned by an adult.

After Rita turned eighteen, she was allowed to visit the homes of her brothers and sisters, who, having settled into arranged marriages, moved to various suburbs in the county. Rita's beauty was not lost on her parents, but they expected that like her sisters before her, she would marry young and live a life of quiet servitude.

The first suitor Rita's parents chose was named Derek. The son of fellow church members, Derek had blond hair and green eyes that Rita recognized although she had never spoken a word to him. The plan was to introduce the potential couple at the upcoming church picnic.

Rita was excited at the prospect of talking to an actual boy who was not a relative of hers. But what on earth would she say to him that he would be interested in hearing? Rita wrung her hands as her family members took turns counseling her about appropriate female-male conversation and behavior. Her stomach fluttered. She felt as if she were about to rocket to a faraway planet.

"Don't talk about yourself, Rita. You can ask questions about him. Then just listen and smile," her sister advised. Rita listened, smiling.

"And make sure your legs are crossed at all times," another sister said.

"No bright colors," her mother added. "We'll go through your closet and pick out a long skirt tonight."

"That'll be easy," Rita said. "All I have are long skirts."

That night, Rita's mind was doing somersaults, and so was her stomach. What would Derek wear? How many inches taller would he be than she? Would he smell of cinnamon or bleach? Hopefully, his teeth would not be crooked and yellow like her angry father's were. Hopefully, Derek would be nothing like her father. Hopefully, he would whisk her away from all this.

Rita knew that at eighteen, she was legally entitled to leave home and never return. But the fact was, she had no marketable skills. Chances were, her ability to churn butter and harvest wheat wouldn't get her far.

She suffered through a fitful sleep, bolting awake every hour or so, unsure of the time since no clocks were allowed in her room. In the morning, the roosters called to her, and up she stood. It was time to start getting ready for her first ever date. She grinned, rolling over the word in her mind: date, date, date.

She pulled on the clothes that had been laid on her chair just before, unannounced as usual, her mother and older sister opened the door and walked in. Privacy was a privilege that no one in the house enjoyed. These were not her ladies in waiting. They were in charge, and Rita was under their control.

Rita had hoped to braid her hair, but her mother and sister each pushed one of her shoulders into a chair. Then they took up hairbrushes and pins and set to work parting her hair down the middle. They twisted it against her temples then collected the back into a bun and pinned it behind her head.

"Here you are," her mother said at last, handing her a white lace bonnet.

Rita smiled through her disappointment. A bonnet and a bun, she thought, wishing she could spend the day in bed. Rita had never spent a day in bed in her life.

Waiting out the morning was difficult. Just the thought of

locking eyes with blond Derek made Rita's pulse race. Finally, it was time to walk to church. Her leather shoes collected dust from the unpaved road as she made her way toward the spot where she knew he was waiting.

Accompanied by an entourage, Derek and Rita met with awkward smiles. Under too many watchful eyes, they exchanged pleasantries. And so it was. Three times a week for a month they sat in each other's company conversing about butter, wheat, bonnets and scripture with straight postures and shy voices.

Rita was bored to death. He was good-looking, yes, but that vacuous smile — the same one she had spent her own life perfecting — made her think he might be a robot. There was nothing warm about Derek.

After one month, the couple moved to the next stage in their relationship. They were given permission to walk by themselves. It was late summer. The flowers were in bloom. The couple walked, mute, down a dusty road at the boundary of a field and then turned a corner.

"You don't have to keep walking with your head down," Derek said. "No one can see us." He grinned sideways at her and she noticed for the first time that his teeth were straight.

Rita grinned back. So Derek was, in fact, human. And not only that. He had a personality. Devilish. And kind.

"Still trying to figure out if you're infected or not," he said next.

Rita looked at him, puzzled. "Infected?"

"Most of you girls don't know where your ass is," he said, still smiling as if she knew exactly what he meant.

"I'm sorry?" she said. "What's an ass?"

He laughed. "Never mind."

The more Rita saw of Derek, the more she grew to like him. In two weeks, she had learned more about the world than she had in nearly twenty years. It was time to share with Derek her dark secret. She wanted to escape this tired, lonely place. And soon.

Now that her parents were quite certain that their daughter was soon to be betrothed, they eased up a little. One night, after a family meal, Derek and Rita bid everyone good night. It was time for their customary end of evening walk. Out of range, the lovers groped one another, undoing bows and strings and clasps. Minutes later, they were tying their clothes, and Derek handed Rita a flask.

"Try this," he said. "It's vodka, but don't take too much or you'll give us away."

Rita had heard of vodka, the clear liquid that looked like water but had mysterious power. She grabbed the flask and tilted it into her mouth. A serious warmth enveloped her for the second time that night. She liked the feeling and sipped again and again. She stood up too fast, and immediately sat down on the ground. Her brain felt soft. She giggled. Derek helped her to her feet and without touching, they trekked back.

While walking, a terrible itch started in Rita's feet and legs. She arrived back at the picnic table, scratching.

"What's wrong, Rita?" her mother asked.

"I must have been bitten," she said, sitting down, rubbing her toes. "My feet feel like they're exploding."

As soon as they arrived home, Rita raced upstairs and pulled off her clothes. Large purple welts marked her feet and legs. Feeling light-headed, Rita collapsed onto her bed. Generally reluctant to seek medical help, her family tried the standard poultice approach. Not only was the smell awful, but Rita's condition seemed to worsen, as her breathing came out in shreds.

"Okay, let's go," her father said, giving up. He bundled his daughter into the truck and drove to the local hospital.

The nurse took Rita's vitals, and they didn't look good. "BP 60/40. Heart rate 120. She's wheezing. Looks like anaphylaxis."

Soon, Rita was in the resuscitation room. As the rash spread along the girl's body, so did the worry that she may be in the midst of a life-threatening allergic reaction.

An intravenous was deftly inserted. Fifty milligrams of diphenhydramine and Zantac were injected, preceded by 0.5 cc. of intramuscular epinephrine.

Rita's abdomen suddenly swelled. When the doctor touched the lower part of her belly, she screamed. But why? Could the sex with Derek have caused God to punish her? Rita feared. Could she be pregnant? Too sick to respond to questions, Rita was in no condition to help the doctors do their job. Whatever happened next would be God's will.

The radiologist examined the abdominal X-rays and ruled out an obstruction. But as Rita's stomach continued to grow, the surgeon worried that maybe there was an infection brewing inside of her. To explore, he conducted a laparotomy. But other than swollen loops of bowel and fluid, he could find nothing abnormal. And yet fluid filled her abdominal cavity fast from her swollen tissues.

Rita was wheeled to the ICU, and she stayed in hospital for the next two months. A series of medical complications and millions of dollars of care later, no cause for her allergic reaction was discovered.

Months later, Rita saw her family doctor for a follow-up examination. It was there that she decided to ask the question that had plagued her since that fateful night. First swearing the doctor to secrecy, she asked whether it was possible that the vodka she had drunk for the first time that night might have caused her illness. She didn't really think so, having heard of many adults who regularly drank alcohol, but the question had nagged her all the same.

And she was right. The doctor explained that alcohol is indeed a rare cause of allergic reactions. Minor effects include headaches, nasal congestion and skin rashes, symptoms which tend to be ignored depending on their severity. But many alcoholic beverages contain potential allergens such as yeast and artificial flavors, as well as rye, barley, malt and hops.

To find out whether Rita was allergic to the vodka, the doctor sent her to the Drug Safety Clinic. And lo and behold, testing revealed that an alcohol (ethanol) allergy was the culprit for her life-threatening anaphylactic reaction.

From then on, Rita refused to drink alcohol — even a sip of champagne at her wedding to Derek was off-limits. But every time she visited her parents' farm, she was sure to take a secret toke of hashish from a stash the couple kept in the glove box of their station wagon. They saved it for just such special occasions.

SELF-PRESERVATION

27

The stench was almost unbearable but despite it, Dr. Williams
kept working. With expert hands, she filleted the fresh corpse
in preparation for the final gut. She placed the scalpel on the
tray then held her breath.

Thirty minutes ago, when she first stepped into the
morgue, she had noticed an odor that was stronger than usual.
Chalking it up to the fact that many bodies had made their
way through the room in a week and some were clearly past
their due date, she had dismissed the smell as nothing out of
the ordinary. Perhaps when yesterday's putrefying body was
discovered in an apartment a week after death, some over-
zealous attendant had gone trigger-happy with preservative.
But the longer Dr. Williams worked, the clearer it became.
There were two distinct odors in the morgue today. One was

the unmistakable smell of death, which was familiar to her nostrils. It was a mixture of waste and necrosis, putrid and stale. The second smelled like too much formaldehyde.

As fumes filled her lungs, Dr. Williams feared a formaldehyde spill had poisoned the morgue. She tried to hold her breath. But as she worked on the new body, the smell grew stronger. And now there were tears in her eyes, blurring her vision and attacking her focus. There was nothing left to do but abort the procedure and release the toxic spill alarm. Immediately, all vents roared to life and the few staff members in the lab vacated the sterile room under flashing red lights and a droning wail.

A couple of weeks earlier, across town, Allan was busy cleaning cages and checking on the welfare of the animals at the Brightsgrove Veterinary Clinic. Growing up, Allan had never pictured himself a veterinary assistant. All along, he had dreamed of being the hotshot vet himself. After all, he loved all creatures. But after squeaking through high school with a report card full of Cs and Ds, he had no choice but to set his career sights lower.

Dogs, cats, rabbits and sometimes rodents occupied the wire cages lining the walls. Regrettably, Allan rarely came in contact with farm animals. Located in suburbia, the clinic was small, and it was the larger clinics that had space to house and care for horses and cows. Allan perked up when someone brought in a snake, but the doctor never knew exactly how to treat it. The X-rays were cool, though.

In Allan's opinion, only wackos brought in rodents. And there were lots of those in these parts. He marveled at how people became so attached to rats, mice, guinea pigs, hamsters and gerbils that they were willing to fork over loads of cash trying desperately to prologue their pets' short lives. What did they hope to gain with all that money? An extra week of life with their pet rat? It was, frankly, unethical to waste valuable time and medical resources on rodents. But hell, he took home a paycheck regardless of which animals benefited.

Allan had reasons for working the night shift. First, he could steal ketamine, a drug used to anesthetize animals before surgery. Allan had discovered the drug at a rave, where some kids shot it into their veins, but most rolled it with tobacco and pot and dragged it into their lungs before puffing out the bitter stench in rings. His friend, Geoff, had pointed out that the stuff was often found in veterinary clinics, much to Allan's delight.

The next day, Allan asked to work the night shift for the first time, and he had been doing so ever since. The drug was easy to find and a joy to smoke. Allan loved the out-of-body experience and hallucinations it produced, allowing him to lie back and simply watch for hours on end.

Then, one morning, Allan fumbled for the phone. He had smoked a lot of ketamine last night and he was still fuzzy. Being woken by the phone was hell but since it hardly ever rang, he had never considered taking it off the hook before bed. He picked up the receiver and grunted.

"Allan, this is Dr. Stillwater. I was hoping you could come in a bit earlier tonight. I need to review a few things and go over your quarterly job performance. Okay?"

"Sure," Allan whispered. "Be in at 11:30." Wasn't it too early for his quarterly review? Maybe this drug was messing with his memory. He rolled over and snoozed for another few hours. Eventually, at dinnertime, he pulled himself up.

Allan entered the clinic greeted by the smell of wet fur, then by Dr. Stillwater and two police detectives. Busted. Dr. Stillwater reminded Allan that despite his long drug record, he had wanted to give the young assistant a second chance in the work world. The doctor explained that he had been watching the clinic's ketamine supply drop each night. He was, frankly, disappointed in Allan's show of weak character.

Allan threw up his hands. He was addicted to the stuff. There really was no way to hide it. Not then, and not now.

Jobless and unable to make bail, Allan languished in jail for two weeks before a trial date was set. The fact that he had stolen jars of drugs from his employer was not in dispute. He was, however, able to convince the judge that it was all for his personal pleasure, and that he never had any intention of dealing the drug to others.

Back at the morgue, Dr. Williams pulled on the new ultra shield biohazard suit. It was she who had suggested that the hospital purchase the fully encapsulated suits instead of the cheaper tactical/military ones. According to the product insert, the suit had been successfully tested to protect against a list of 230 different chemicals.

She zipped up against what was, most likely, a simple formalin spill, went to the cupboard, and verified that all specimen bottles were tightly closed. Surprisingly, she found all formaldehyde dispensers sealed with no evidence of drips or leaks. Now this was strange indeed. Where was that stench coming from? There were but a few sources of formaldehyde in the lab.

A frustrated Dr. Williams stripped off her biohazard suit. Donning an N95 mask, she returned to the autopsy room. She followed the stink to the southern end, a large sterile square with the capacity for a hundred bodies. This was the spot where she had been in the midst of cutting when she had sounded the alarm.

Dr. Williams approached the corpse, concluding that it must be the source of the smell. Had the technician inadvertently sprayed the body with formaldehyde before the autopsy? It would be out of the ordinary, but she called in the tech anyway. He assured her that no, he hadn't yet met this particular corpse. Still, the doctor was quite sure that the smell pre-existed her postmortem examination.

Confused, Dr. Williams continued to examine the body. She removed the sternum then saw that several organs were abnormally discolored for a fresh specimen. The grayish discoloration was in fact typical of a fixative, such as formalin or formaldehyde. She sliced open the stomach, then stepped back as the stench powered into the room. The gastric contents were soaked. The pharynx, esophagus and stomach were inflamed and corroded. Dr. Williams shook her head and called police.

During Allan's employment at the clinic, he stole more than just ketamine. Figuring that one day he'd be caught, he needed a stash of stuff to sell for drugs. So when he spotted a one-gallon jar of thirty-seven percent formalin lying around in an unlocked cabinet, he pinched it. True, he had no idea what the stuff was for. But it sure did make him feel powerful to own it.

At room temperature, formaldehyde is a gas. The solution is called formalin. An excellent disinfectant, formalin kills just about everything. It is used as a preservative and as part of compounds that eradicate warts. Because it preserves, or fixes, living or dead tissue, it is a mainstay of the embalming industry.

Dr. Williams learned that the decedent was found in his apartment, and although his corpse was one week old, it was in surprisingly excellent shape. As it turned out, with his source of ketamine cut off, Allan had no reason to live. So he drank the formalin, carefully placed the empty bottle beneath the sink, and lay down on his bed to die. In the end, he simply had no sense of self-preservation.

NYLONS AND LIGATURES
AND SNARES — OH MY!

28

According to her boyfriend, Marta collapsed after a typical night of excessive partying. Janusz explained to police that she had stormed out in a drunken state. First, she had scoured the house for more whiskey, and she was furious when she came up dry. By then, she was so smashed that she could hardly find the front door, he said.

Some time later, Janusz became worried, and he left the house to look for her, he said. He himself was somewhat drunk and even a little stoned, so the details were blurry. He couldn't remember how long she had been outside before he got up to check on her. He might even have fallen asleep on the couch first. But he did recall being relieved that there was no sound of a car engine after she left. At least she couldn't get into any real trouble, he had figured.

But Janusz was wrong. As soon as he stepped off the porch, he explained, he saw Marta lying there. She was sprawled, facedown, on the lawn.

"I thought she had passed out," Marta's boyfriend told the detective. "But when I shouted in her ear and she just lay there, I rolled her over."

That's when Janusz found himself staring into unblinking eyes. Even then, he thought his girlfriend was just hammered. He picked her up, carried her inside to the couch and covered her, gently, with a blanket.

"I thought she just needed to sleep it off," he said.

Janusz explained how he had sat in the chair opposite the couch, and fell asleep himself. When he woke, and Marta hadn't moved, he touched her skin. She felt cold and stiff. In a daze, he said that he sat in that chair in the dark for a few hours more, horror spreading like a cancer through his blood.

Finally, he dialed for an ambulance.

Paramedics arrived at the decrepit shack with the wrap-around porch. They stepped over and around empty beer bottles on their way to the front door. Marta was still lying on the couch. In the kitchen, Janusz had his head in his hands.

Marta's face was tomato red, but she looked comfortable on the pillow, her body beneath a fuzzy blanket. Finding no sign of injury, the medics took thirty minutes to confirm that Marta was dead. First, they had to follow protocol and patch in to the emergency room physician. As they examined the body, Janusz stood mute, a cigarette lodged between shaky fingers.

Although the medics found nothing suspicious at the scene, save for a loop of hair beside the couch, they called in the forensics team to investigate. Soon, Janusz was sitting in the back seat of the police cruiser, making his way to the station for interrogation. Once there, he repeated his story again and again, and new details kept emerging.

"I called police when I was sure she wasn't waking up. She had asthma you know. I told her she shouldn't smoke. I think that's what killed her, the asthma." Janusz dragged on the butt of yet another cigarette. "I didn't expect her to die. How does someone just die like that?" He looked at the detectives, dry eyes pleading.

The detectives answered by continuing to pepper the boyfriend with questions. "Why didn't you call right away? Immediately?"

"I don't know," Janusz said, shrugging. "I was drunk."

"And how long did you wait to call?"

"I told you, I waited an hour or so," Janusz replied. "I don't remember."

"Why did you move her again?"

"Because I thought she would be more comfortable on the couch. Where was I going to put her?" Janusz asked.

Finally, the questions slowed. Detective Scott, the fat one, gave the suspicious looking boyfriend a long, cold stare.

"Wait here, Mr. Adamicz," he said, using both hands on the table to hoist himself up. "I'll have a quick chat with my partner, and I'll be back with another cup of java for you. I think you could use it, buddy." With that, the two detectives left the interrogation room.

"Seems a bit jumpy, no?" Detective Larsen, the skinny one, said, absently stirring his coffee with a plastic fork. "His live-in lady dies and he just doesn't seem that broken up. It doesn't make sense. He finds her outside and carries her to the couch. Wouldn't most people call it in and leave the body? Do you believe he didn't know she was dead?"

"He was drunk, so anything's possible," Scott said. "And you know as well as I do, we can't hold him unless we charge him."

With no obvious signs of suspicious activity, they had no choice but to wait for the coroner's report. Maybe the gal simply overdosed, Scott thought. The boyfriend seemed shady but sometimes, a language barrier made people seem shadier than they were.

Detective Larsen reentered the interrogation room where Janusz sat on a folding chair, his head against the wall. A glass ashtray that seemed to be coughing up butts sat on the table. The detective grabbed the other folding chair, twirled it around and sat down, his chest against its spine. He glared at Janusz. A few seconds passed. Janusz stared at the wall.

"You're free to go, Mr. Adamicz," the detective said. "We'd like you to stay in the city, though. We'll get back to you as soon as the coroner completes his report. Sorry for your loss."

After a decade in homicide, Larsen suspected there was more here than met the eye, but it was always better for a suspect to believe he was free and clear. Less of a flight risk — especially with immigrants. Was there even an extradition treaty with Poland? He'd have to check.

Janusz looked relieved as he filed out of the room ahead of the detectives. His tobacco stink veered down the corridor, stepped inside the elevator, and vanished.

As in every case, the coroner was looking for evidence of murder. Here lay a well-nourished middle-aged woman with horrible dentition and long dirty hair. Her face was congested and dotted with pinpoint hemorrhages called petechiae under her skin, appearing as tiny red dots. Interestingly, the distribution of the dots was around the face and upper neck, and there were more hemorrhages in the mucosa of her mouth. The coroner was suspicious. There was a clear demarcation mid-neck where the petechiae suddenly stopped.

Finding the rest of the autopsy unremarkable, the coroner collected fluid samples for toxicology and phoned the detectives.

Like savvy lawyers, detectives prefer to know the answers to questions they ask of suspects. When Scott and Larsen went after Janusz a second time, they were pretty sure they knew what his answers would be; the trick was in getting him to say them out loud.

Janusz hadn't bothered to shave since they saw him last. From his smell, he hadn't bothered to shower either. Even though Janusz couldn't seem to still his shaky hands, Larsen asked if he wanted a coffee. The boyfriend shook his head. He hadn't slept in days because his lids refused to close for fear that the ugly scene would replay, yet again, in his dreams. The detectives didn't even have to speak. Janusz started to cry. Between hiccups and sniffles, he talked.

"I didn't mean to kill her, I swear it!" he blurted.

"It's okay, just tell us what happened," Larsen said, helping him.

"She wouldn't shut up. Yelling, screaming like a freak. I told her to quiet down and did she listen? No."

"So what'd you do?" Scott asked, intrigued.

"I just grabbed her head to shut her up and she kept squirming and struggling, like a fish on a hook. I just wanted to keep her quiet," he said, tapping his foot on the floor, fast.

The detectives were nodding.

"I wrapped her hair around her throat, just to keep her quiet. I didn't twist and pull it for long, I swear," he pleaded. "Just a minute or so, and then she went limp so I carried her inside. She wouldn't wake up. I didn't mean to kill her." He hung his head. Again, he began to sniffle. "She was always so proud of her long hair!"

The cause of death was asphyxiation from strangulation. Although ligature strangulation is a common method of homicide, this was the first reported case that involved using the victim's own hair as the weapon.

Janusz was charged with second degree murder, and while awaiting trial, he too was found strangled. Perhaps as a way to avenge his girlfriend's murder, share her pain or ease his conscience, he had committed suicide. On his feet were shoes without laces — the same laces that were found twisted and then knotted around his neck.

SCREWED

29

Like his dad, Eric had always been good with his hands. And since school just wasn't his bag, he needed those hands to earn a living.

At just sixteen, Eric gave up on grammar and arithmetic, and plunged like an anchor straight out of eleventh grade into unemployment. It wasn't that he didn't understand the work; it was just that he didn't see how calculus or economics or poetry was going to help him wire a family room or drywall a basement. A skilled linebacker, even with the recent knee injuries that slowed him down, he was sure going to miss high school sports, though, especially football.

When, at dinner one night, Eric informed his parents that he was leaving school for good, there were no protests. In fact, his dad's eyebrows quivered with excitement. Now he could pull his son into the family construction biz early. Just think of all the equipment he could buy with the cash he would save in free labor.

Eric was a fast learner, and by the time he hit twenty, he was ready to earn more money by choosing a specialty rather than just working as a jack-of-all-trades. The fact was, he was tired of mixing paint and hauling bricks. So he focused on securing his electrician license. After a three-year apprenticeship, the bare minimum, Eric was on track to becoming a master or even journeyman in the field.

Eric was smart enough to know that contracting work was typically secured by word of mouth. Do a good job and it will lead to five more, his dad always said. Early in his electrician career, Eric was hungry, so he would work pretty much any job just to build his reputation. With his dad's connections, he was hired to rewire and replace an old circuit box with a breaker to accommodate a new kitchen in an old suburban house. Eric estimated that the job would take just a few days of solo work to complete.

Atop a small stepladder, Eric screwed in a light fixture bracket. His knee was aching. Two arthroscopies and torn cartilage had left him with a creaky knee joint that felt decades older than it was. Even with the powerful knee brace he wore for support, Eric still winced when climbing ladders. But doing so was part of the job.

"Eric, any chance I can get you to install a ceiling fan in the master bedroom before you head out?" It was Jamie, the contractor who employed him.

"No problem. I'll get my tools from the truck." Actually,

it was a problem. It was getting late and Eric's stomach was growling like a tiger. But saying no was not an option if he wanted more recommendations.

Eric's knee buckled as he stepped down from the ladder, a screwdriver clenched between his teeth. He twisted sideways and lost his balance. It was a short fall, just four feet onto a plush carpet. Saved.

The thump brought Jamie in from the downstairs kitchen. Eric was conscious. Phew. The last thing Jamie needed was a claim from workers' compensation.

But the young man was whimpering. "I can't move my legs," Eric said, and then blood spouted from his mouth onto the rug. Within a minute, he passed out but the bleeding from his mouth continued, staining the rug in a growing circle.

Jamie stood and watched. He had dialed 911 but now felt helpless, having been told by the operator not to touch Eric. But it was frightening to see his man lose so much blood. To keep himself occupied, Jamie collected the blood-soaked tools scattered beneath the ladder and ran them under cold water in the sink.

Right away, the medics saw the source of the blood was Eric's mouth but they could not make the bleeding stop. So they gave up trying and worked to slide a tube down his throat to establish an airway.

In the hospital resuscitation room, an hour of intense effort was going nowhere. Eric's mouth was a faucet of blood, and the trauma surgeons were growing more and more frustrated. The patient's blood pressure and heart rate were so unstable that he could not be moved out of the emergency department for imaging.

The team placed Foley catheters in Eric's nostrils and inflated them in hopes of staving off a possible sinus bleed. They drilled burr holes into his skull. Both an ear nose and throat surgeon and a gastroenterologist scoped Eric. But with the field of vision obscured by the gush of pumping blood, no one could find and stop its source.

Finally, Eric bled to death. It was a rare case inside the emergency department where doctors can usually stem the flow of blood in young patients.

The next day, Eric's body arrived in the morgue for autopsy. The pathologist had a hard time prying open his mouth. Despite multiple transfusions, the young man's heart and lungs were emptied of blood.

The pathologist examined Eric's teeth, one by one. As noted by the medics and emergency room staff, the left central and lateral incisor and canine had been ripped out. Careful inspection of the mouth revealed an oval hole in the hard palate nearly an inch long and a half-inch wide. Closer inspection identified a penetrating injury through the base of the skull. The right internal carotid artery had a hole in it. The length of the wound from the hard palate into the brain was nearly four inches.

The pathologist checked the cranial X-rays to ensure that there was no bullet in Eric's skull — particularly since there was no exit wound at the back of his head.

Jamie answered the door of his home to find two policemen standing on the porch.

"Can we come in and have a word about yesterday?" asked the stockier of the two.

Jamie led the men into the dining room where the three sat.

"Can you tell us again exactly what happened when you heard the thud?" one of the cops asked. He needed to find out what object had penetrated Eric's mouth, carotid artery and brain.

"I heard a crash," Jamie began. "It wasn't loud, but I rushed upstairs anyway, and there was Eric, lying on the carpet with blood gushing from his mouth. He was dazed, eyes closed and he muttered that he couldn't move his legs. He didn't say anything else. That was it. I called the ambulance the minute I saw the blood. There was so much blood."

Jamie's voice was shaky. He couldn't get around the feeling that Eric's death was his fault. He had been the one to get the guy the last job he'd ever have. He had asked him to install the fan and doing so had killed the kid.

"Okay, listen," a cop said, leaning close to Jamie. He spoke slowly. "Did you notice or do anything else? Think. I need you to tell us anything and everything. Don't leave out any detail — even if it seems irrelevant."

Jamie thought for a moment. "Well, after I called 911, I cleaned some bloody tools. Under the water, in the sink."

"What tools?" the stocky cop asked.

"Well, there was a screwdriver, a Phillips, which was lying beside Eric. He must have dropped it when he fell, and then there were some other tools around, too. They were all full of blood."

"Where's that screwdriver now?" one of the cops asked.

"After I washed the tools, I returned them all to the kid's

toolbox. I felt so helpless. I didn't know what else to do." Jamie dropped his head into his hands. Tears were coming again.

"Where's that toolbox?"

"Still at the house," Jamie replied. "No one really wants to go back there right now. We kind of temporarily put a hold on the work, you know. Out of respect."

The policemen thanked Jamie and returned to the scene where they promptly retrieved the screwdriver from Eric's toolbox. Then they drove to the hospital and explained to the pathologist what they had learned.

The pathologist found that the thin steel shaft measured nearly four inches to the molded plastic hilt. Inserting the screwdriver into Eric's brain was like finishing a jigsaw puzzle. A perfect fit. The pathologist constructed a theory. Eric had descended the ladder, as he had no doubt done hundreds of times before, with the screwdriver in his mouth. When he lost his balance, the shaft of the tool drove straight through his hard palate, lacerated the right internal carotid injury and passed into his brain. The plastic handle shot forward knocking out three teeth. The pathologist surmised that Eric must have used all of his strength to pull the screwdriver from his mouth before he collapsed and Jamie arrived on the scene.

There was no way to tell whether leaving the screwdriver intact would have saved the young man's life. The general rule, however, is to leave an impaling object in place until it can be properly removed in an emergency room. Otherwise, as in this case, and in some reported cases of hard palate impalement involving pencils, bicycle handlebars and crowbars — usually found in kids — the victim is in danger of bleeding to death.

FECAL MATTERS

30

Some occupations can make you rich, even if you have no edu-cation or experience. That's because there are jobs out there that no one in his right mind would choose to take on without a financial incentive. If the price is right, some people will do anything.

Devon was fortunate enough to have one of those jobs. Free of the constraints of a college degree or even a high school diploma, Devon happily hauled sludge. At first, when he saw the ad seeking employees in the paper, he had no idea what the word even meant. Sludge is, in fact, a general term for a soupy mixture of solids and liquids separated from one another, like meatballs in tomato sauce or clams in chowder.

Devon didn't haul just any sludge, though. He wasn't lucky enough to transport vats of chowder or meatball sauce.

He trucked the standard by which all sludge is measured: human waste. What most people don't know is that the stuff we deposit in our toilets every day has a natural tendency to separate. In the tony world of urine and poop, sludge is the sewage at the bottom of the barrel.

So Devon spent his days hauling putrefied raw sludge, the accumulated sediment of sewage left to sit for a couple of hours. It's not a pretty sight, and one that most of us would prefer not to picture. After hundreds of thousands of people stand and squat their waste into the toilet, it meanders through increasingly large pipes beneath our homes and sidewalks, and travels, forgotten, to sewage treatment plants where it settles in special tanks reinforced to prevent leakage. Within the tanks, bacteria accelerates the decomposition process of putrefaction and liquefaction, which reduces the volume of the messy mix.

Sick as it may sound, Devon prided himself on the fact that he was a sludge expert. In fact, he knew more about human sludge than most college graduates. But it was knowledge that he didn't exactly race to share with his family, friends or dates.

In a 4000-gallon truck, Devon hauled digested excrement to landfills. But since margins in the waste hauling world were narrow, it was difficult for the company Devon worked for to invest in the newest, more modern tanker trunks. As the hydraulic system raised the container on the truck diagonally, the open hatch allowed the contents to slide out the back, propelled by gravity. It was similar in concept to the manner in which the sludge left its original owner: dumped.

It was a filthy job, which would have been made more fun

if Devon could ride in the fancy tanker. But at least all he had to touch was one button to raise the container. There were no vacuum suctions or shovels, like on some of the old models. Still, it was hard to maintain a sterile environment when you were spending eight hours straight around sewage.

Driving the muck was easy. It was loading and unloading the truck that was dirty work, in spite of a healthy stock of company issued coveralls, gloves and masks. Three times a day, five days a week, Devon dumped sludge into a large man-made landfill. The site, safely removed from populated areas, measured nearly a mile wide and thirty feet deep.

Devon was concerned about the toll his employment took on his social life. He divulged his occupation to only his closest friends but was careful to describe himself merely as a truck driver when meeting new people. He couldn't help but worry about his future. These secrets somehow squeezed their way out, he knew. The question was: How could he find a woman and start a family when his job involved hauling excrement? And even if he was lucky enough to land an understanding wife, what would he tell his kids?

He could hear the playground talk already:

"What does your daddy do?"

"He's an accountant. What about your daddy?"

"Oh, he's a shit trucker."

The kindergarten teacher wasn't likely to invite him to speak on career day — that was for sure.

Devon was feeling anxious about where all this sludge hauling was leading him when he arrived at the landfill at the same time as Craig, a fellow driver who had hauled for most of his working life, just over thirty years. If Devon continued along the path he was on, he worried that one day, he might end up exactly like Craig — potbellied, smelly and alone.

Carefully, Devon backed the truck to the edge of the ditch, angling it for a smooth transit of excrement into the landfill depths. He activated the hydraulics and the loader creaked upwards. Exiting the cab of his vehicle, he shuddered at the thought of spending twenty-five more years hauling slimy sludge.

"Heya Craig!" he called. "Late haul today?" Craig should have done his business and been gone an hour ago.

"Last one of the week!" Craig called over the rumble. Craig pointed at Devon's truck. "Hey! Your hatch looks stuck again!"

Looking up at the motionless near-diagonal container, Devon cursed. This truck was a lemon and he'd been stuck with it for too many months now. How many times had the company mechanics assured him that it had been repaired? Too many to count. What did they care, he thought now, sizzling with frustration. I'm the one out in this field of shit. Maybe if they had to find a way to dislodge human waste every time the door got stuck, they would work a little harder on a permanent fix. Better yet, he thought, maybe I should dump my load on management's front door.

"Shit!" Devon called out. "Third time this week! How hard is it to fix a bloody steel door?"

Craig said nothing. Instead, he hustled over to the cab of his truck and disappeared. The last thing he wanted to do was help Devon again. His own job was hard enough.

On his way to the back of the truck, Devon cursed the malfunctioning hatch. It was rusted and bent, and the company was too cheap to fork over for a new door. So each and every time it got stuck, it fell to Devon to fix it, which meant getting his hands dirty. He hated touching his load. Even in his own washroom, Devon went through half a roll of two-ply toilet paper with every seating.

As he had many times before, Devon wondered whether this was all worth it. Did he really need the extra cash this job paid? Standing outside thousands of gallons of human sludge, unable to cajole it into a giant pit, he made a decision at last. This was Devon's last haul. He would rather flip burgers or stock shelves at midnight. Screw the money.

But first, he had a problem to overcome. Devon pulled the sledgehammer from the truck and began hammering at the back door. Nothing happened. He kept pounding away, letting his anger fuel his swings as they raged against the steel. Pound after pound, Devon smacked that hammer until his shoulder started to ache, and still, he kept pounding. He was so angry, he would never, ever stop. Soon, he began cursing and shouting with every swing, smashing the truck, the company, the mechanics, the job.

Then, with one final mighty smack, the hatch opened with a pop, and a fraction of a second later, an avalanche of shit roared down on Devon, carrying him like an ocean current to the edge of the landfill. Craig rushed from his truck to help his friend. But unable to withstand the pull, Devon teetered on the edge for but a moment before vanishing, as the sludge continued to pour forth with thunderous force.

Devon tried to cry out but when he opened his mouth, the excrement slammed to the back of his throat. Craig saw his friend bob to the top of the slurry before he was buried beneath it.

Recovering the body was a joint effort. Craig, the fire department, marine unit and forensic team all helped. Everyone donned expensive environmental suits except for Craig. He was used to the feel and smell of the stuff.

After an hour of dredging from an aluminum boat launched onto the lake of waste, the would-be rescuers finally snagged Devon's body from the bottom of the pit. It was the most disgusting recovery effort any of them had ever heard of, let alone been involved in. After the episode, the boat they used had to be disinfected with ammonia and it sat immersed in antibacterial solution for over a week.

The postmortem was conducted outside the morgue building in the surrounding courtyard. Even to the seasoned pathology workers, the stench emanating from Devon's corpse was just plain intolerable.

After reading the police report, the pathologist knew she had to make this quick. She took tissue and fluid samples to confirm that Devon had not been under the influence of alcohol or drugs, then she noted that sludge not only covered his entire body but was also clogging his mouth, pharynx and lungs. There was no doubt. Death was determined to be by accidental asphyxiation. Devon had met his death by choking on the waste that so many nameless bodies had innocently flushed down the toilet, never to be thought of again.

IT'S ONLY A FLESH WOUND

31

After number six, Ryan had lost count. Along with a few of his buddies, he had been celebrating at the off-campus pub since his last exam of the semester. That was ten hours and countless shots ago. He had aced the organic chemistry final, that was for sure. He had better have aced it, after putting his life on hold for three months.

Ryan wasn't particularly moved by organic chemistry. Or biology, or physics, or biochem, or any of the subjects he was required to take to make it into med school. But he would study his brains dry nonetheless.

With three years of university under his belt and a 3.95 GPA to show for it, Ryan had a good chance of getting in. He wasn't a shoe-in, though. Not even with a near perfect academic record. His GPA was good but might not be good enough. The fact was, there were legions of equally hardworking first and second generation Chinese and South East Asian achievers to compete with these days, and they were making it tough to bag one of the two hundred spots in medical school. Let's face it, there were 2,000 applicants. Still, Ryan was a confident twenty-year-old.

He worked hard and he partied hard. In equal measure. When it came to drinking, he was a star. He could tolerate more alcohol than any guy he knew. His liver enzymes were part of a well-oiled machine, he figured, breaking down alcohol with increasing efficiency. A lesser man would surely be in the emergency room by now.

It was almost 2 a.m. and Colonel Nathan's was about to close. After draining each glass, Ryan had peeled a fiver off his roll of bills and tossed it onto the bar. Beers cost $4.60 each, so Ryan would drink those now, until his stash of fives was gone. He never left Colonel Nathan's with money. He knew his limit.

Tonight, though, Ryan felt sick. He was slurring and stumbling, but made it home to the front porch leaving a trail of vomit behind him. He climbed the front steps then fell.

Ryan shared the rented house with two roommates, Clayton and Pitch. Pitch was Simon Pitchowski, a skinny kid with a prematurely receding hairline who was known for his whiny voice. Pitch was popular. He was the friend you could count on when you locked yourself out or got your girl pregnant or feared you may have messed up and failed an exam.

Now in the midst of pursuing a degree in anthropology, Pitch had spent his childhood dreaming of excavating ancient ruins in the Middle East. He had just returned from a volunteer dig in the Golan Heights in Israel, arriving at the house around the same time that Ryan answered the final question by shading the bubble with his standard number two pencil on the Scantron chemistry exam. Still jet-lagged, Pitch had been sleeping for hours when he was awakened by the sound of banging on the front door.

Impatient with a drunken sense of the passage of time, Ryan lumbered to the side of the two-story Victorian home and pounded on the window. Still half asleep, Pitch was shuffling to the nine-foot front door when he jumped from the sound of a loud smash. He froze in the hallway. Then the banging started on the front door again.

Pitch was annoyed. Finally, he unlocked the front door only to find his friend Ryan standing on the stoop, his shirt soaked red. He was gripping his forearm where blood seemed to be spurting from a cut in the rhythm of his heartbeat — one and two and three and four.

Pitch was no med student. An anthropology major, he was dumbfounded by the sight of blood and the implications of the fountain spouting from his buddy's arm were lost on him. Besides, he was still half asleep.

"Shit, Ry!" cried Pitch. "What the hell?"

"Fergot my key," Ryan slurred. "Broke the window with my fist." He laughed, evilly, then his eyes went dim. "Jush need ta banage this bleeding. It's jush a flesh wound and I gotta lie down. Gotta sleep, man." He looked up at Pitch with a goofy smile. "Gooda seeya, Pish."

"Ryan, do you have to drink so much every time you finish a goddamn exam?" Pitch was yelling, as if his friend might not be able to understand him at normal volume. "I mean, you've got enough exams to take you to middle age! You're gonna end up a freakin' alcoholic!"

Pitch ran to the kitchen for a dish towel but when he returned to the door, Ryan was gone. He followed the trail of blood to the bathroom where Ryan was sitting on the closed toilet lid, his head resting on the counter top. He was snoring. Pitch lifted Ryan's arm and wrapped it in the towel. The bleeding seemed to be letting up.

"Bedtime, kid," he said. "You're cleaning up this mess tomorrow. Not me."

Ryan used all his effort to raise his head. He mumbled something incoherent, his eyes reduced to two slits in his sweaty face. With his rescue effort complete, Pitch hit the sack. He was dreaming as soon as his head hit the pillow.

The following morning, Pitch awoke at 7 a.m., feeling stale. He stretched and yawned and rubbed crust from his eyes. Sitting on the edge of his bed, he looked at his hands. There were dried flecks of blood on his fingers and traces on his sheets, too.

Damn. He'd be cleaning up Ryan's mess again. Enough was enough. Cursing, he strode to his roommate's room and knocked on the door. He was tired of acting like an unpaid servant in this house and he sure as hell wasn't on drunken blood duty. It may be early, and his friend may be hungover, but Ryan was getting up and scrubbing that blood off his fresh sheets now. If he had to kick Ryan out of bed early, tough.

The bedroom door was open a crack. Pitch pushed it and yelled at the bed. "Get up, you lazy shit! Who told you to drink so much? Go and clean the bloody house! Looks like someone was stabbed here last night!"

Ryan's room was a hurricane of science texts, papers, clothes and empty food boxes. He had yet to clear the detritus from months of intensive studying. But there was no Ryan.

Maybe he passed out on the couch, Pitch thought. Heading downstairs, he saw more blood in the hall than he remembered. Pools of purple and red clots led from the front door to the bathroom. The walls were smeared in crimson streaks. Frightened, Pitch headed for the family room couch. It too was empty.

That's when Pitch felt a knot of panic in his belly. There really was a lot of blood. It was scaring him. He followed the parade of purplish red to the bathroom door and nudged it open. There was Ryan, still sitting on that closed toilet lid, sleeping with his head on the sink counter. He was exactly where Pitch had left him.

"Ryan, man. Get up," Pitch whispered in Ryan's ear but his pal didn't move.

"Ryan?" Pitch called louder, his voice at its whiniest. "Get up, man!"

Ryan remained still. Pitch touched his friend's cheek. It was cold. He was like an island in a sea of blood.

Had he not been so drunk, Ryan, the would-be med student, would have known exactly what was happening to him. Unlike Pitch, Ryan was well aware that veins don't squirt; they trickle and ooze. Arteries, on the other hand, spurt, and only deep lacerations spout like a fountain from the forearm. The radial and ulnar arteries supply blood to the forearm and hand and these vessels course deeply beneath the layers of muscles.

The body's main artery, the aorta, branches into the sub-clavian artery, which becomes the axillary then the brachial artery before separating into the ulnar and radial arteries at the elbow. At Ryan's forearm, a shard of glass from the broken window had completely transsected his brachial artery. The laceration was deep — so deep that while both boys slept, Ryan had silently bled to death.

Quite appropriately, the coroner determined that the death was due to accidental exsanguinations from misadventure. But now Ryan's adventures and misadventures had come to an end.

THE CATCH OF THE DAY

32

*Gary, dad to four, grandpa of nine, loved fishing. A retired fire-*fighter, he earned a generous pension that had bought a small property on Lake Bluegill, just a two-hour drive from Ottawa, Ontario, with its own little town just twenty minutes south. There was nothing that tickled Gary more than casting reels off the dock with friends and family. He loved to brag about how he taught each of his grandkids the joy of a hook, a dew worm and a sunset.

Of course not all of his grandkids shared Gary's passion for fishing. Eve, the oldest, and Lily, her younger sister, abhorred the practice. The first time Eve watched her grandfather remove the hook, along with most of the gastrointestinal tract of his catch, she vowed never to eat another dead animal.

"It's the circle of life, Gramps," Eve explained. "You can't kill living things for sport without upsetting your Reiki balance. There's bad karma around your dock, I can feel it."

Gary would just chuckle and tousle Eve's mop of red hair. She was such a little firecracker.

Lily avoided all discussions about fish. Between raw fish guts strewn on the dock and her sister Eve's foreboding psychic predictions, she learned to avoid heading out to the dock if Gramps had a fishing rod over his shoulder. The solitude of cottage life allowed Lily to play her clarinet. A virtuoso, Lily had secured a place with the National Youth Orchestra, wowing the faculty with her perfect rendition of "Flight of the Bumblebee."

It was late one August morning. Gary had been awake for hours. The coffee was perking, the eggs were sizzling, and Grandpa Gary was flipping pancakes as his kids packed for the trip back to the city.

"Drive safe!" Gary called to his family as they piled into their van to hit the road after breakfast. Alternating between swatting mosquitoes and waving goodbye, he watched them pull out of the gravel driveway.

"Well, Joan, looks like we're on our own for the night," Gary said to his wife, playfully slapping her backside. "Should we head back first thing tomorrow?"

"Sure thing, love," she replied. "I'm taking a dip. Joining me?"

"No thanks," Gary said, watching her climb the stone stairs leading into the cottage. He would rather fish in the lake than swim in it. "I'll take a shot at catching lunch," he said, heading for the dock. "See you in an hour."

Gary made his way down to the boathouse, pushed open the wood door, and breathed in the smell of fresh cedar and rodent piss. He plucked his fishing box from the shelf. Gary's boat, a 20-foot Cobalt, floated from a hoist on the ceiling. Maybe I'll cruise the lake, anchor, and cast a lure, he thought. But cruising was no match for lounging in a wide wooden Muskoka chair with a six-pack of Premium Ale while he fished off the dock. He grabbed a worm from a Styrofoam container. Pinching it between his forefinger and thumb, he speared the guts, looping it around the hook. The worm wriggled as it oozed from the puncture wounds.

After casting his line thirty feet out, Gary took a seat and chugged his second bottle of beer. The sun high in the sky, he nodded off, only to be woken by a tug on the line. Dazed, he pulled hard, and reeled in his catch with more force than he needed. He could tell that whatever was on the other end didn't weigh much.

Gary had fished the lake for decades. He'd throw the small ones back. But sometimes the hook had pierced the poor creature so deeply that when he tried to remove the steel barb with pliers, he killed it. That's when he'd imagine his granddaughter chirping in his ear, "It's one thing to end its life for food, but for sport, well, that's just sad."

It took a few moments for the five-inch sunfish to come shaking above the waterline. Gary yanked and the fish flopped on the planks of the deck, gasping in the humid air. Gary's back creaked as he leaned over and grasped its body. It seemed hardly worth the effort. The hook was caught in the upper lip. Using pliers, he wrestled it free. Then he held up the wriggling fish, and shadowed against the setting sun, it suddenly flipped, flew from Gary's hand and landed headfirst in his open mouth.

Shocked, Gary staggered back and tried to cough the fish out. As he flailed backwards, he slipped on the wet dock and fell. The thud interrupted the morning silence. Sudden searing pain and a sickly crack told him he had just fractured his hip. Struggling and panicked, Gary reached inside his mouth to finger out the fish but could not get hold of its slippery tail. He desperately tried to get up, but he couldn't move. Unable to shout for help, his arms flailed spasmodically, reminiscent of both the worm and the fish as they were speared.

In the meantime, Joan waded out of the water and carefully toweled herself off on the narrow strip of sand. She pushed one of the heavy Muskoka chairs into the sunlight, squished into the seat, and prepared to start an old paperback that a long forgotten guest had left after a weekend visit. Looking toward the dock, she saw her husband. Why was he passed out? Was he drunk this early in the day?

Joan sighed and heaved herself out of her chair, muttering. It wasn't easy for a woman of her girth to get in and out of chairs.

"Gary!" she shouted, trying to save herself the fifty-foot walk to rouse her husband. "Gary?" But when he didn't answer, she resigned herself to the interruption and trekked over. After forty years, she was still looking after the guy.

As soon as she neared him, it was clear that this was no regular drunken snooze. Her husband was lying on his back, one leg grotesquely twisted. His eyes were open. Fearing a heart attack or stroke, she knelt on the wood and started CPR. Immediately, she gagged. There was a putrid smell in her husband's mouth. Confused that she was unable to force even a wisp of lifesaving air into her husband's lungs, Joan gave up, and waddled as fast as her thick legs could carry her to the phone to dial 911.

When the paramedics arrived, Gary was cold, and his face and lips were blue. He had no heartbeat. Still, the medics feverishly worked on his lifeless body, inserting an intravenous line and barking orders to one another in hopes of a miraculous rescue.

"Intubate him!" one medic ordered. They knew the man was gone, but with his panicked wife watching, they felt obligated to show their best attempt at saving her husband's life.

One medic grabbed the laryngoscope. As he pried open Gary's mouth with its long curved blade, he spotted a silvery tail. "There's a damn fish in his mouth obstructing his airway!" he shouted. "Quick! Grab the McGill's!"

Within seconds, the McGill forceps were passed from hand to hand. The medic inserted the forceps over the laryngoscope and snagged the sunfish's tail. Then he started CPR again, rhythmically pumping and blowing but Gary lay still. They loaded his body onto the stretcher and into the rear of the ambulance.

Unwilling to face his widow, the medics transported the corpse to the hospital where two things were clear: Both Gary and the fish were dead and never again would those medics be able to stomach tuna sandwiches for lunch.

INSIDE OUT

33

After fifteen years of reconstructing thousands of accident scenes, Bentley was tired. Kneeling over yet another corpse, he looked up at the clear sky and concluded that weather conditions could not have factored into this fresh kill. He also decided that this was his final day on the job. He simply could not wake up to one more dead body.

Bentley had come to despise his job. The hatred was slow to develop. It took years of insomnia and irritability, a nasty divorce, and escalating alcohol abuse to get him to this point. He felt as if he had been withdrawing from caffeine for over a decade.

Antonio sat in the back of the police car. At least he wasn't handcuffed, he thought, relieved. Not that there was any reason to cuff him. After all, no crime had been committed.

He had plowed into the jogger at forty miles an hour, just ten over the speed limit. He knew the guy was dead the moment he felt flesh hit steel and the airbag pillowed his chest. The poor man flew through the air, twisting like a kite in the wind, until he landed on his head a good fifty feet away. It was like watching a slow motion video, Antonio thought now.

He had, of course, hit the brake hard. There was nothing else he could do. What he didn't do was rush out of his car. Through the cracked windshield, Antonio could see the motionless man lying in the middle of the road. He picked up his phone and dialed emergency services. Raw all over, he waited until he heard sirens heralding the approach of an ambulance. Only six minutes had elapsed since the collision.

After determining the jogger was dead, the medics appeared at Antonio's window to offer assistance. He waved them off. He wouldn't talk until he had to. Aloud, he cursed the jogger. What kind of jerk runs into traffic when there are perfectly safe sidewalks?

Officer Fitch appeared at his window. Antonio knew him well, so he pressed the button, letting it slide halfway down.

"Sorry, man," he said. "I can't give any statements without my lawyer."

He picked up his phone again. This time he dialed Solomons, of Solomons & Hayden, Barristers and Solicitors. He left a message on the answering machine. It was still early. S & H was a respectable downtown law firm — not one of those ambulance chasers. If anyone could get him out of this mess, it was a professional like Solomons.

Detective Bentley had been briefed by Officer Fitch. The

case was straightforward. It was dawn and still dark when on his way to work at the Division, Officer Antonio Cabrera hit a jogger dumb enough to be running on the road — wearing black shorts and a black T-shirt with black socks and shoes, no less.

Of course, that didn't explain how the guy had been impaled through the mouth by a white pole.

The medics saw it first. It looked as if the jogger had already been intubated with an endotracheal tube in an attempt to resuscitate him, but that was impossible. They had been the first to arrive on the scene, and there had been no one around. Even the driver had remained in the vehicle. And yet there it was.

Antonio's car was a Honda Odyssey van. The bumper, having sprung from the body of the vehicle, lay on the ground a few feet away. A semicircular impression fitting a human body was evident in the hood. The windshield had splintered but remained intact. Bloodstains spattered the metal and glass.

Kneeling over the corpse, Bentley examined the body with gloved hands. It was still warm. Well-built male. Forty-five-ish. His shoes lay about fifty yards away but his iPod earbuds still hung from his neck. The head was twisted and bruising and fractures were apparent on his arms, legs, and ribs.

What had this man landed on? It looked as if he had died halfway through eating a white bloodstained snake. Through fifteen years and thousands of accidents, Bentley had seen all manner of deaths, from domestic assaults to jumpers. And yet, he had never seen anyone land openmouthed on some kind of white pole that he couldn't instantly identify.

Bentley beelined for Antonio's car. They had been two

cops who worked on the same floor, and they were friends. Bentley pulled open the car door, but before he had a chance to say a word, Antonio put up his hand.

"Lawyer only," he said. "Sorry, Ben."

Bentley had always wondered where on earth his parents had found the gall to name him Ben. It seemed like a lame joke, like Kris Kristofferson, Henry Fitzhenry or Johnnie Johnson. He was, believe it or not, Ben Bentley. The only way to get around the teasing had been to lift weights, and become a cop.

"Just trying to figure out what he landed on, Tony," Bentley said. "He's got some kind of whitish cylindrical tube or pole attached to his mouth. I can't figure out if he was eating something while jogging or there was something at the side of the road."

Antonio knew Bentley was simply trying to understand what had happened. But rules were rules and having been in this business long enough, he knew enough to follow those.

"Lawyer," he said, shutting the door. He had no idea what Bentley was talking about. All the more reason to wait for Solomons, and to sit quietly in his car at least until the cor-oner arrived. It wasn't routine to bring him in to the accident site but these were unusual circumstances.

Thirty minutes later, Dr. Lewis pulled up. Nearly retired and always disheveled, he exited his car, plopped his fedora onto his head and surveyed the body. Meanwhile, a smile stretched across Bentley's face. He felt giddy. This was his last case, ever. He might as well enjoy the final scene.

Dr. Lewis glanced at the white snake. "It's his cord," he said simply. And with that, he turned and walked back to his car. He hadn't even kneeled over the body.

The pole looked fleshy because it was. The impact of the crash had been so severe that it ripped the man's second and third cervical vertebrae, transected the spinal cord and lower portion of the brainstem (the medulla), and propelled his spinal cord through his mouth, making it appear as if he had swallowed something. In fact, the direction was opposite to what it seemed. The cord was exiting, not entering, the man's body.

Bentley was still leaning over the corpse, smiling. Who would have thought that his last ever accident reconstruction would be a first for him? He stood up and strolled to his car wondering how he would spend tomorrow after handing in his last accident report. One thing was for certain: he would then, officially, be living among the living.

LET'S GET SMASHED

34

"Be there @ 6:30 to get table," the email read.

Ah, Saturday night. Dan looked forward to it all week, every week. It was a break from hauling garbage.

A career as a sanitation engineer was surprisingly lucrative. It not only paid the bills; it also provided a fat pension Dan could feed off when he retired. He considered himself lucky. A unionized municipal worker, Dan was employed for life, and paid more then he deserved for his lack of effort. After a five-day work week, during which he put in a mere twenty hours of true labor, he was itching to party. For him, weekends were for guzzling at the bar and cheering for his team in a drunken stupor. He could hardly wait.

Dan always got an early start. To save a few bucks, he slammed back a few glasses of rum with a splash of Coke before veering out to the subway station. For the past eight years, the drink had been his drug of choice, ever since his dad had let him sip when he was fourteen. He was still hooked.

The Trash Boys, as they referred to themselves, met every Saturday between 6:30 and 7 p.m. at Strauss' Bar and Grill. Since they all came from different corners of the city, no one ever drove. Besides, they would all be so blitzed by last call that cars would be hard to find, let alone recognize. Subway was the safe route, for sure, even though it took twice as long.

Feeling high, Dan locked the door of his apartment and aimed for the station. It was a fifteen-minute walk. The air was cold and the trees looked starved. When Dan arrived at the subway platform, he was alone. Heralded by a blast of wind, the subway car arrived with a screech. He boarded the train and feeling giddy, fell into a seat as the subway lurched forward.

Ten minutes later, he exited at St. Patrick station. He was almost there. The bar was all noise. The earliest patrons had settled into leather booths lining the perimeter while the rest stood jockeying for the bartender's eye. Dan surveyed the crowd and spotted Noah and Jarrett tucked in a booth at the back.

"Lucky for us tonight!" Dan yelled. He squeezed in beside Noah and took a swig from the beer bottle sitting on the table.

"Get your own bloody beer!" shouted Noah. "Sip mine again and I'll crack it over your head!"

Dan motioned to the waitress but knew from experience it was a lost cause. He glanced at the jumble at the bar. He was tipsy from the rum but knew the odds: If a strong buzz feels good then imagine how a stronger buzz will feel. Swaying,

Dan pushed his way through the crowd, ignoring the insults peppering him. Finally, he spotted his favorite bartender and waved. "Four beer and four glasses," he slurred.

"Coming up," the bartender said, motioning to a waitress and sending Dan stumbling his way back to the booth.

When the final two members of the Trash Boys, Aaron and Hunter, arrived, the five friends got busy guzzling beer and shouting at the football game on the screen. Hours passed as they blurred into drunkenness. Dan had tripped twice on the way to the washroom and on his third visit, elbowed a young woman sipping an apple martini beside her boyfriend at the bar. She stepped back but not in time. Her drink landed on her silk blouse with a splash.

"Hey, Asshole!" the boyfriend shouted. Lost in the thump of music and oblivious to his own actions, Dan kept walking, focused on the toilet sign. Suddenly, a hand gripped his shoulder and flung him backward against two other guys. Dan shouted and within moments, Noah, Jarrett, Aaron and Hunter were slicing the crowd, pushing anyone in their path, making their way to their friend. They were all large men, tattooed and muscular.

Fueled by alcohol, punches flew in every direction. The bouncers, even larger than the sanitation engineers, separated the groups and stood in the middle of the fracas. They pointed Dan and his entourage toward the door. It was not the first time they had dealt with this particular group of brawny men. These guys seemed to have a penchant for bar fighting.

"And we bid you good night," Dan slurred, bowing to the crowd. It was time to move on to the next watering hole.

But before the group could make their way out, a wineglass was launched from across the bar. It sailed through the air and smashed against the right side of Dan's neck.

Immediately, a cherry red spray jetted across the hardwood. His neck pulsated, and Dan fell to the floor with a thump. A bouncer jumped down and used his hands to apply pressure to Dan's bleeding neck. But in just over a minute, it was all over. Dan was dead.

We humans have about five liters of blood pulsing through our blood vessels. The body pumps that amount each minute to produce what is known as a person's cardiac output. In this case, Dan's heart spewed his entire cardiac output onto the floor of the bar as soon as the glass shard slit his carotid artery. The bouncers could not contain the crowd as they ran in a current toward the exits, slipping and sliding on fresh blood along the way. The only patrons left were Dan's friends, shocked and drunk, in the empty bar.

There were no witnesses left to identify the thrower of the glass. The police interrogated each member of the sanitation posse but they were too intoxicated to provide the details necessary to kick-start an investigation. While one friend claimed the murderer wore a black shirt, another insisted it was a gray hoodie. Depending whom you asked, he had blond, black or even red hair. He may or may not have worn glasses that were either wire-rimmed or thickly framed. Thankfully for the girl's boyfriend, there were no surveillance cameras to assist police.

But one question remained. How had the wineglass severed Dan's artery?

There were shards of glass lying on the floor beside the

body. The homicide squad bagged the evidence and the coroner bagged Dan. There were no fingerprints on the largest shards of glass; however, the glass's rim was broken. That jagged rim acted like a knife, slicing straight through Dan's neck. For poor Dan, it all came down to the worst possible luck.

HITTING THE JACKPOT

35

Ever since Jerome took his first steps, he had been throwing balls and swinging bats. At twenty-two, he was partway through his third year of a baseball scholarship at Northern Alabama University. But Jerome wasn't all about sports. He was a biochemistry major, and he worked hard to maintain at least a 3.7 GPA.

Still, Jerome was banking on his star athlete status to catapult him into the field of dentistry. He had heard that the admissions committee slobbered over students who excelled at extracurricular activities. Thankfully, his reputation as a champ was well known around campus.

For awhile, Jerome had flirted with the idea of abandoning university to go professional in baseball but ultimately decided it was a gamble he wasn't prepared to take.

The likelihood of establishing a career as a pro athlete was too remote to abandon his studies. He wanted a sure thing, a job that would provide him with a stable financial future.

Everyone knew that in teeth, the real moneymaker was orthodontics, but there were only a few positions available each year. And no doubt, the cream of the crop would apply. But first things first, Jerome thought.

Still, although he focused hard on schoolwork, there was no denying that on the baseball diamond, Jerome sparkled. For three seasons in a row, his batting average led the team. A killer in the batting box, he had no fear of stepping straight into ninety-two miles per hour fastballs. Even more impressive, Jerome's power ranked him among the top ten home run hitters in collegiate baseball in the country. On the field, he was all about the adrenaline rush of hitting balls.

After a month of nonstop studying, Jerome found himself in the home stretch of final exams. Physics, a requisite course for dental school admission, was his last hurdle. Even the most basic equations stumped the star player. Calculating $F = ma$ just didn't come naturally to his brain. And $KE = \frac{1}{2} mv2$ drove him crazy.

He steered his mind around the questions, trying to follow. "If a car was traveling at 60 miles per hour at an 80 degree angle . . ." Jerome's thoughts swerved. He was tired of stupid what-ifs, and anyway, he had a plan that, if executed properly, would propel him straight to an A.

Everyone knew that undergrad multiple choice questions on physics exams were recycled. The same ones showed up every three to five years. Those lazy professors never bothered to change them. It was their fault, Jerome thought. If they were going to underestimate the industriousness of their students, well, they should be duped. And those students, having demonstrated foresight, should reap the rewards.

In fact, if Jerome was clever enough to find a way to acquire fifteen years' worth of physics exam questions, then he deserved an A, he decided. He may not have any idea what the answers meant, but he set to work committing each and every one to memory. Sixty-eight kilojoules, 100 meter/second, 11.4 volts. Now that was hard work.

The Friday morning of the big exam, Jerome shivered. The fact that he had written hundreds of exams did nothing to calm his nerves. At the gym entrance, he flashed his photo and slid his fingerprint over the scanner. Rows and rows of chairs were arranged in a grid pattern. Taking his assigned seat, Jerome waited for the starting bell. His undershirt was already wet. The test was three hours long.

Jerome finished in half the time, and after spinning his pencil around his fingers for a bit, he handed in his paper an hour early. Most of the answers slid from his memory to the page, and he took wild stabs at the few questions that looked new. Should be enough for an A, he concluded on his way out of the gym, smiling toward the weekend ahead.

Jerome set out to spend that night hunting for action, and he didn't have to look far. There were always babes hoping to hook up with a jock. He called a couple of Oriental beauties who had texted him from the bleachers during his last game and went on to bed both in his apartment. After the act, he kicked the girls out, then wandered to an off-campus party, first stopping at the dorm room of his buddy Jake.

Jerome always felt safe heading out in the night with Jake because his friend always packed a firearm. A few years ago, Jake had been robbed at gunpoint, and since then, he had felt the need to protect himself. With Jake around, they could always defend themselves against drunken partygoers. There wasn't a bar brawl they could lose.

Not that Jerome needed to worry. He hadn't had a drink in five years. After a couple of meaningless fights as a teen, one of which left a chunk of tooth embedded in his knuckle and another that landed him in hospital for four weeks of intravenous antibiotics to combat a serious infection, he had sworn off alcohol.

At the frat house, Jerome looked around the party. It was the usual: girls strutting around half naked, guys swaying with beer. "Boring! Let's cut out!" Jerome yelled, pointing to the door.

Jake nodded and they left.

"Where to?" Jake asked, patting his front pocket. He was making sure his 0.22 caliber was safely settled in.

"Let's head back," Jerome said. "Gotta rest up for next week's games."

Their strides matching, the guys headed back to Jerome's bachelor pad. Once inside, Jerome put on some tunes and Jake lit a joint. Before long, both boys were flying high on the couch.

Jake pulled out his pistol and emptied all six chambers, except one.

He looked sideways at Jerome. "Feeling lucky?" he asked.

They both sputtered with laughter. Jake pointed the gun to his own temple. Then, with a click, he squeezed the trigger.

Jerome's mouth hung open. "You're crazy, man. What do you think you're doing? You just had a 16.7% chance of dying." He sucked at physics, but hell, he knew his formulas.

Jake chuckled, spun the chamber and handed it to his buddy. "You're up, dude. Feeling lucky?"

Stoned, Jerome looked at the gun for a long, lazy minute. Oh, what the hell. He pointed it at himself, then at his friend, and in a flash, put the gun to his own head. No bang, no explosion, just a small metallic click. That was easy.

The little game of Russian roulette played out. Jake and Jerome, for reasons neither knew, passed the gun back and forth, like kids taking turns sharing a toy. They had pretty much forgotten that there was a round of live ammunition waiting to splatter gray and white brain matter all over the 400 square feet of living space.

Jake pressed his luck. On his fourth try, the metal click indicated another stroke of good fortune.

"Okay, wrap it up, dude," he said to Jerome, dropping the weapon into his buddy's palm for one last round. "Your turn and we're done."

The collegiate athlete, who was shooting for dentistry with — as it would turn out — a 3.8 GPA, and refused alcohol lest it mess with his judgment, pulled the trigger. It was his last conscious act. The gun fired and Jerome's body pitched forward, blood drenching the couch in seconds.

In general, high-risk behavior is associated with lack of

parental oversight, poor self-esteem and trouble in school. Peer pressures, family problems, drug and alcohol abuse and sexual activity are typical precipitants. The overwhelming majority of those who engage in high-risk behaviors — from autoerotica to Russian roulette to racing cars — are men.

Like Jerome, most Russian roulette victims are playing the game under the influence of drugs or alcohol. But unlike this case, most resulting deaths are not purely accidental. Studies show that they occur mostly in men who have had a history of psychiatric struggles, including depression. And since Russian roulette is known as one of the most extreme forms of high-risk behavior, some classify the losers of the game as victims of suicide.

HEAT OF THE MOMENT

36

Yvon was on the run. He stuffed as much as he could fit into a sturdy knapsack, closed the door to his apartment for the last time and strode the thirty blocks to the train station. The pockets of his camouflage pants bulged with bills he had saved for just such an emergency.

Now that Yvon had been positively identified, his face must be flashing on every late night broadcast in the country. That damn storage unit he had rented years earlier was no help. Way back then, it hadn't occurred to him to use fake ID. Dumb move. An hour had passed since the attack and his mind was clear enough to make his getaway.

Making his way to the train, his head aching, Yvon felt for the laceration on his scalp. Beneath his winter hat and thick head of black hair, the wound ran deep. He knew he hadn't lost too much blood. Luckily, he had a first aid kit in his apartment and had used the needle and thread to stitch the wound.

He was, of course, disgusted with his behavior. It wasn't the sexual assaults — which he had been performing with reasonable skill since high school. He was proud of the fact that he was meticulous in his planning and execution. What other predator had included monthly surveillance and checklists in his stalking? Yes, his attacks were an art form, scientifically rendered.

What disgusted him was the fact that he had been sloppy enough to get caught. For two years, he had evaded the hunt of the dozen or so uneducated Keystone cops assigned to his case. And now he had done himself in. He had tripped himself up. Just like that, Yvon's bravado was gone. After he got himself out of this, after he found a way to blend back into the crowded, faceless world, he would have to punish himself.

Yvon picked up the pace and jogged toward the station and a train ticket that would whisk him to the far end of the country. He made a mental note to purchase a return fare although he had no intention of ever coming back.

The morning had started like so many others. He awoke to find her facedown, tied to the bed in the storage room he had rented and converted into living quarters. She was still cute in her pajamas. Yvon never assaulted his women within twenty-four hours of capture. He waited to let the fear boil and then simmer for awhile. But this morning, he awoke later than expected. The alarm had been set for 13:00 so when his eyes opened to the sight of the LCD display signaling 15:12, he panicked. He had just eighteen minutes to get to the factory.

In twelve years, he had never been late for work. He could kill her without having sex first. He could suppress the urge to screw her. But then he would be deviating from the norm, and that would not do. Arriving late at work, though, would jeopardize his job, so he had no choice. He would have to leave her, work the night shift, return to his apartment to shower, and then come back to the storage unit. He loved her terror. It kept him focused. In the meantime, the deviation from his routine might actually be an opportunity, he thought. He took an orange juicebox from the small fridge and forced a straw into her mouth. He would feed her only fluids. That way, she would lose weight and feel nice and skinny.

He went through his dress ritual. Hair, teeth, panties, nylons, socks, boots, uniform. He glimpsed the mirror on the way out. It was just a short walk to the factory. He was reaching for the doorknob when he heard a sound. It was just before the lamp hit him.

Shocked, Yvon crumpled to the floor. Lying on his side, eyes gaping, he saw her legs running toward the doorway. He reached out and grabbed for the pajamas, tripping her. Their eyes locked. She kicked him in the head, right where the lamp had hit. Grimacing, he let go and watched her run out the door and into the daylight. He could not for the life of him figure out how she had slipped the restraints.

Yvon's army training kicked in. He knew what he had to do and waiting for a herd of police to cuff him was not in his plans. Still groggy, he went straight to his apartment. Life as he knew it was over, and it was time to plan for the future.

There was only one possibility. The rope he had used to

restrain her was too old. He had used it too many times on too many girls and the bitch had worked on it with her teeth all night. It was the only way. From now on, he would need a new modus operandi. From now on, he would cuff each girl to the bed.

He was only a few blocks from the station when he checked his watch. He should have enough of a head start to be safely on his way before the cops got their house in order. It would take hours before they would finish their coffee and donuts and get on the road. The lazy butts. Yvon had inside info, having been a cop for two and a half years himself. That was before he was fired.

Outside the train station, the August Nevada heat was suffocating. Dripping wet, Yvon downed a box of orange juice and tossed the carton in the bin. It was mid-afternoon, a perfect time to escape.

Having picked his destination, Yvon waited in line at the ticket booth. He tapped his foot as everyone inched forward. He felt sweat beading on his brow. But when it splattered onto the floor, he saw that it was not in fact sweat, but blood. Cool and calm, Yvon left the line for the washroom. He locked himself inside a stall, sat on the toilet and dabbed his wound, careful not to wipe any clots that may have formed.

He heard the bathroom door swish open followed by a female shout. "Police! Come out with your hands in the air!"

This was the second time today that shock ripped up his spine and his police training kicked in. Yvon opened the stall door and faced two cops, a man and a woman. Palms up, he strode toward them.

"On the ground!" yelled the man. He was standing only four feet in front of Yvon, his gun drawn. Yvon knew the drill. He turned and knelt, his back to the policemen and laced his hands behind his head. As the cop moved forward, one hand grabbing Yvon's hands and the other reaching for cuffs, Yvon turned and made his move.

Shock flickered in the cop's eyes. The policewoman wasn't taking any chances with her gun. It was too easy to shoot your fellow cop in a struggle. So instead, she jumped into the fray and tried to grab Yvon, who was already sprawled on the floor straddled by the policeman. Even with two of them, though, they could not pin his arms as he twisted with the ease of a contortionist.

Displaying what seemed like superhuman strength, Yvon was only partially restrained. Any part of his body that was not immobilized writhed and thrashed. After ten minutes of fighting like a mad wrestler, Yvon had punched and kicked the policewoman unconscious. He was, for the moment, free.

Feeling light-headed, the fugitive sprinted for the door and pushed it open, only to welcome three more cops inside. They were alerted to his whereabouts by the shouts and grunts echoing from the washroom. All at once, Yvon was on the ground. His limbs flailing beneath the weight of the police, he would never surrender. But he was outnumbered. Five minutes later, he emerged with arms and legs cuffed and a mouth that was clenched and spitting. He refused to relax. He would fight to the death.

The cops forced Yvon forward. Just as he stepped outside the washroom, he began shaking for two full minutes.

Without sympathy, the cops dragged him into the sun where a mob was waiting on the sidewalk. That's where Yvon went limp. Hundreds of eyes witnessed his collapse. Unable to hide Yvon's obviously dire state, an option they would have preferred, the police called an ambulance to attend to their barely breathing detainee.

The medics arrived and found Yvon unconscious, hypotensive and markedly tachycardic. Assuming a head injury had caused his collapse, the paramedic inserted an intravenous and started fluid resuscitation. The cops insisted on riding inside the ambulance as it transported Yvon to hospital. Handcuffs locked all four of his limbs to the stretcher, but with crazies like this guy, you just never knew.

In the emergency department, police flanked the comatose patient as the physician reviewed the officer's story. Presuming head trauma, he ordered an emergency CAT scan. But before the patient could be transferred, he suffered a cardiac arrest. The medics pumped his chest for thirty minutes, trying to resuscitate him.

During the efforts to save Yvon's life, a nurse noted that his body temperature measured 41.5 degrees Celsius, a full five degrees above normal. Somehow, Yvon had become critically hyperthermic. While he had in fact suffered a head injury when the lamp hit him, Yvon did not die from the blow.

The pathologist found cuts and bruises all over the dead man's face and body. His heart was dilated and his lungs ballooned with bloody fluid. All organs, including the liver, brain and skeletal muscles, showed the effects of severe hyperthermia, a condition that results when the body absorbs more heat than it dissipates. Overexertion on a hot day is often the cause.

Yvon not only lost blood, but he also made the mistake of sprinting thirty blocks wearing a warm, wool cap. Then, his sweaty struggle with police generated too much heat for his body to get rid of in time. In effect, he became a human torch without any means to cool off. He overheated, one could say.

STEAK AND LEGS

37

Clarice was worried. Her neighbor Wayne was a fixture on the street. So it was strange that she hadn't seen him in three days. His yard was like an immaculate nursery: coiffed bushes and a blanket of green lawn, not a weed in sight. Toward the back, Wayne had planted small bunches of purple and white perennials and a couple of fruit trees that were still too young to yield a harvest. It just wasn't like him to be AWOL.

Clarice took to spying. She would peel back the satin living room drapes just enough to peek out in hopes of catching any sign of Wayne. She had been carrying on with the man for the better part of a year and the truth was, she desperately missed their daily trysts.

The pattern had been well practiced. After dinner, her husband, Edward, retired to his study with a cognac in one hand and a cigar in the other. As soon as his nose was buried in the *Wall Street Journal*, Clarice would shout that she was heading outside to tidy the garden, mow the lawn or sweep out that messy shed once and for all. When she realized she was running out of yard work excuses, she hit the hardware store and loaded her cart with garden gnomes, bird feeders, birdbaths and anything else she could think to stick on her lawn. The bottom line was this: the more garden decorations she planted outside, the more reasons she had to slip out of the house and into the arms of her sexy neighbor.

They always met in the shed that stood on the northeast corner of her property. It was easy for Wayne to access the door from his yard since there was no fence between the two homes. Instead, the yards were delineated by a row of bushes, easy to hop.

They always did it the same way, she standing with her back to him. Clarice took to wearing low-cut sundresses in the middle of fall. The more she thought about it now, the wider she spread the curtains. With twenty years between them, Clarice harbored no fantasies of a future with Wayne. Still, it just wasn't like him to skip their nightly rendezvous.

For the past three evenings, at 6:15 p.m. sharp, she had stood alone in the shed for fifteen long minutes, waiting for the door to swing open. When it didn't, she made her way back to the house, her chest tight with worry.

Finally, she couldn't take it anymore. With Edward safely at work, Clarice marched up Wayne's driveway and knocked on the front door. It opened and there stood Wayne Junior. Clarice had not seen the young man in many months. He used to live with his father — up until his hospitalization, that is. Hopefully now, he was cured.

Clarice stepped inside the house and Wayne Junior closed the door behind her. His face was like a mask, his mouth barely moving as he spoke right through her. He was a human robot, she thought, a cyborg.

"Dad's not in," the young man droned. "He took a fishing trip with some friends. He won't be back for weeks."

That was strange, Clarice thought. She hadn't even asked about his father's whereabouts and already Wayne Junior was serving up information. Goosebumps crawling up her arms, Clarice mumbled something about the garden and said a cheery goodbye before rushing back to her house. There was one thing she knew for certain. Wayne hated fish.

Now Clarice was practically living in the living room. She parked a chair beside the curtains and obsessively kept watch over the house next door. It took only two days for her to reach quiet hysterics. While her husband went about his days oblivious to her plight, Clarice could not get the headline out of her brain: *Widower murdered by mentally ill son.* She thought of the neat shed straddling their lawns. It had been such a perfect arrangement. She was going to miss Wayne behind her.

On the evening of her fifth neighborless day, Clarice couldn't take it for one more second. She picked up the phone, called the police and explained that her neighbor had disappeared.

"He lived alone, Officer," she said, trying to hide the fear in her voice. "His son was released from Glenview Acres only last week and I — well — I think he might have killed his father."

There. It was out. She had said it.

Clarice imagined that Wayne Junior had murdered his father for his neat, perfect bungalow. In her fantasy, she could see Wayne's corpse propped up on the couch watching TV with the same transfixed gaze his son had when he opened the door.

The officer reassured Clarice that he would send over a couple of uniformed cops to investigate. He didn't think much of her story, though. Calls from concerned, paranoid, anxious, delusional and/or lonely neighbors were all too common.

Three hours later, Clarice watched two police officers rap on the door of the house next door. They began to knock harder, then to pound. Then seeing a flash of movement behind the drawn curtains, Officer Leiber thumped the door with his truncheon and barked an order.

"Open the door! We can see you're inside! Open it or we break it down!" The officer's face reddened. He thumped the painted white door again, leaving scuff marks.

"Open up!" Officer Swensky shouted. He kicked the door frame. Resisting the urge to shoot the handle, he pulled out his radio and called for backup.

Within ten minutes, two more cops had joined Leiber and Swensky at the door. Holding a metal battering ram, they called out 1-2-3 before drilling forward. The door flung open.

All four police saw the bloodstains at the same time. They drew their guns and stepped inside the house. In the kitchen, they found Wayne Junior whistling as he prepared dinner. Seemingly deaf to the orders to raise his hands and get down, he shook the pan on the stove. In it was a steak fillet sizzling in oil.

The police took slow steps toward their suspect and prepared to fire. Wayne Junior simply stood like an automaton, flipping and frying, whistling.

The cops forced him to the kitchen floor and handcuffed his wrists as he lay like a rag doll. Swensky twisted off the stove burner and the team of police began their slow walk though the house.

In the fridge, the officers found two human legs and a shoulder. All skin had been expertly sheared off, exposing muscle, tendons and vessels. In the crisper, there was a collection of bags later identified as human organs. In the freezer sat a human pelvis, and inside its cavity were what appeared to be steak fillets. On the kitchen table was a half-eaten steak. There was no side of rice, spaghetti or potatoes anywhere to be found.

In the upstairs bathroom, the tub was filled with crimson water. A butcher knife and a collection of bloodied kitchen knives were clustered together in the bathroom sink.

The officers contacted the homicide squad then removed all animal protein to examine at the morgue.

Reconstruction identified an incomplete human male. According to his fingerprints, it was definitely Wayne. Of the missing pieces, most notable were Wayne's head and brain. When asked about this peculiarity, Wayne Junior just shrugged. He also refused to explain where his father's genitalia had been misplaced.

Mostly, Wayne Junior just shook his head in response to the questions that were fired at him. He did, however, nod when asked if he had murdered his father in a ravenous fit of rage. Apparently, the missing organs had somehow found their way into Wayne Junior's stomach.

After her lover's son was declared not guilty by reason of insanity, and safely committed to an institution for life, Clarice was never the same. From then on, she couldn't help but spend her days peeking out from behind the living room curtains.

Cannibalism derives its name from the Spanish word for the Carib people of the West Indies (*canibalis*) who ate human beings. But cannibalism is not restricted to humans eating humans; the term refers to any animal eating its own kind. Around the world, various tribes have made it a practice to eat their own. In modern times, cannibalism has thrived in parts of Africa during wars in Liberia and Congo.

The book *Alive: The Story of the Andes Survivors* by Piers Paul Read chronicles another modern-day example of cannibalism. The act occurred in 1972 after an air disaster of a Uruguayan Air Force turboprop. The plane crashed in the Andes while carrying a rugby team, a muscular group of men. Of the forty-five people aboard, eighteen died from the crash within eight days. Others succumbed to the harsh mountainous winter, including eight who suffered the added misfortune of an avalanche. The survivors had no choice but to eat the corpses in order to stay alive.

FOOD FOR THOUGHT

38

Warren Chan remembered the first time food started talking to him. He had been sixteen years old, sitting in McDonald's on a leatherette seat full of crumbs when out of nowhere, his burger said, "Eat! Eat now! Eat and be free!"

Warren had looked around, thinking maybe the voice had come from the next table. But then his fries spoke in a voice that was deeper, rumbling. "Time to eeeeaatttt . . ." the fries boomed, ominously. Warren had shaken his head, and as the talking continued, he actually tipped it to the side and smacked his ear, trying to right his brain. When that didn't work, there was nothing left to do but eat the food. That would silence the little buggers.

Soon, all food facing Warren couldn't shut up. And since the only way to deal with the problem was to eat it, Warren was blowing up like a blimp. He'd have to eat, then hightail it to the bathroom, and stick his finger down his throat to eject the food into the toilet.

It worked. Through bulimia, Warren was able to keep his weight stable, and keep his secret from the world. But his eat-purge lifestyle prevented him from joining the workforce like regular folk, so at thirty-eight, he found himself not just lonely, but broke, living off monthly welfare checks.

That income was not enough to buy the pills his psychiatrist prescribed for what was clearly a psychotic illness, though. Thank goodness the state paid for intramuscular depot injections of the antipsychotic drug fluphenazine during monthly visits to the psychiatrist. The jabs alleviated his symptoms somewhat. But Warren hated the dry mouth and appetite loss that were unfortunate side effects. So every once in awhile, he gave himself a break and skipped his doctor's appointment.

Within a week, though, the voices began to taunt him. "Eat!" each potato chip commanded before he popped it into his mouth and crunched it to death. "Eat and be free."

Warren silenced the voices by devouring everything in sight. Chips, pizza, bananas. The type of food was irrelevant. Without his meds, his appetite soared, his taste buds became numb from eating so much so fast, and his food choices were running low. Warren was in the middle of one of his "cycles" as he liked to call them. He had eaten himself to sleep again.

An old blanket hung from the ceiling, shading the apartment's only window. The building shared an alley with a Chinese food restaurant known for its all-you-can-eat buffets.

It was Warren's dream and nightmare, and it was so close, but a dinner of kung pao shrimp and beef in oyster sauce would leave him penniless.

Warren awoke to the buzzing of flies. It took him minutes to realize that he was lying in a pool of undigested vomit. Around him lay six empty boxes of Kraft Dinner, two one-liter bottles of Tahiti punch and three cartons of mostly eaten Krispy Kreme donuts, which he finished off, pronto.

The night came back to him now. Too full to waddle to the washroom, he had not been able to wait. Pink torrents of macaroni and cream-filled sludge had splashed from his gullet onto the linoleum floor. He recalled looking at a bottle of aftershave, wondering what it would taste like going down right before he nodded off. He had only snoozed for a few hours before the flies got to him. The buzzing pounded inside his head.

"I could eat you, Fly," he said, imagining himself gripping the little critter by the wings and swallowing it whole.

Rousing Warren from his dead sleep, the stench assaulted his nostrils. He sat up, nearly slipping on the stinky bits of food flowing in his digestive juices. Then came the voices.

"Feed me!" they implored. "I'm hungry, so hungry!"

Warren slapped his hands over his ears. The more he tried to ignore his voices, the louder they sounded. They seemed to be coming from his sixteen-inch black-and-white TV. Was his favorite movie, Monty Python's *Life of Brian*, playing? No, there was no picture. Only sound. Incessant whining for food.

"Search the cupboards!" the TV commanded. "Search the cupboards and feed!"

Overnight, Warren had transformed into an insect. He

was a giant hissing bug that needed food, only food. He sloshed about the floor, finally righting himself, a bloated sticky beetle. His socks were soaked pink, his hair plastered against his forehead.

"Eat!" the voices shouted, yelling, begging.

That's when Warren saw them. A group of Chinese cooks had made their way into his apartment. They marched in single file, dressed in crisp white outfits, sporting matching Fu Manchu mustaches, holding identical stainless steel butcher knives in the air. The gaggle of cooks jabbered away, while Warren nodded. When had he learned Cantonese? It was amazing! Why, he could understand every word!

"Pork spare ribs. Wonton soup. Steamed rice. Happy meals. Eat."

Never much of a leader, Warren followed the commands. He stood up and marched to the kitchen. Once there, he methodically emptied the cupboards and fridge of every edible item. He opened, he peeled, he unwrapped, sucking back everything within reach. Frozen hot dogs, a jar of pickles, mustard, eggs, peas. When Warren could no longer budge from the weight of all that food inside him, he dropped to the floor and slurped up the vomit.

Lying down, Warren lapsed in and out of consciousness. The gurgling cramps that shot through his belly were nearly loud enough to silence the cacophony of voices in his brain, but still, he ate. Finally, after downing the contents of an entire box of Raisin Bran and gobbling two lemons, skins and all, his cramps cut sharp, forcing him to stop.

Warren's stomach had ballooned. It was so distended that

when he looked down, he couldn't see his legs. He craved relief from the voices, from the pain, from life. But as sick as he felt, Warren craved something else, too. Staring at the ceiling, he pondered the most important question of all: "Where the hell were those gummi worms, anyway?"

At that moment, Warren's stomach and intestines ruptured. Straining against his diaphragm, the jumbled contents of his abdomen exploded into his thoracic cavity, and with murmurs of discontent from his voices echoing around him — "Eat! Swallow! Eat and be free!" — Warren collapsed.

A full week later, the superintendant smelled something sickly coming from Warren's apartment. He held his breath and knocked on the door, then began pounding. Finally, he called police.

Inside the apartment, the stench made it impossible to breathe. No one could enter the scene without wearing Level C body suits. In fact, it took two weeks of scrubbing with bleach before the superintendant could show the place to prospective tenants. He would, of course, keep mum about why it was vacant.

At autopsy, Warren's abdominal cavity was still full of undigested food. What hadn't spilled over remained in his massively dilated stomach and intestines. The pathologist determined that the cause of Warren's death was asphyxia and a ruptured stomach secondary to extreme polyphagia, or overeating.

In some people, the more common conditions of anorexia and bulimia overlap with other "fringe" eating disorders, such as polyphagia, where one can't stop eating. Pica is a condition where the person's uncontrollable appetite is for unusual items such as dirt or ice.

As for Warren, he was done in by a combination of bulimia, polyphagia, and pica, all of it brought on by his untreated psychosis. In the end, he found relief. He was cremated, and his ashes fit inside a small cookie jar. He was smaller than he had ever imagined.

THE NOSE KNOWS

39

Little Atul was sick. He had been a healthy four-year-old just last week, and now the boy was pale and lethargic, his nose dripping blood. His father had no choice but to carry his son all the way to the village nurse in Kalapani.

Atul's father explained to the nurse that it had all started with a nosebleed from both nostrils. Then, over the past two days, the bleed had become a faucet until this morning, when Atul began vomiting blood as well.

The nurse recorded the details of the nosebleed, or epistaxis as she called it, and the bloody vomiting, otherwise known as hematemesis, and she examined the listless boy as he lay on the clinic bed. His brown arms protruded like twigs from the sleeves of his burgundy T-shirt. A few sizes too big, the shirt only amplified Atul's sickly appearance. The nurse was certain the boy was suffering from leukemia, and yet she could find no abnormalities to support her diagnosis. There were no petechiae, or red spots, on Atul's skin. There was no evidence of an enlarged liver or spleen.

Still, the child was obviously very ill. The nurse feared that he might even be in imminent need of a blood transfusion. And since the village clinic lacked the proper facilities to investigate more deeply into the boy's condition, she instructed his frightened parents to arrange a transfer to the main hospital in the city of Abbottabad, twelve kilometers away.

Atul's parents scrounged enough coins to pay a modified taxi to drive them into the city. It took nearly an hour for the Suzuki van to pull up and then the driver idled the car until more passengers filled the van. Only then would he set off. Sick kid or not, he needed the fares.

In the emergency room of the Ayub Teaching Hospital, little Atul was a pitiful sight. He sat scrunched and small between his mom and dad in the crowded triage area overnight, waiting his turn, holding rags to sponge the blood coursing from his nose. Finally, after more than twenty-four hours had passed, Atul's name was called.

In the examining cubicle, a resident doctor appeared. He stuffed gauze up the boy's nostrils to stem the flow. Within seconds, though, the blood soaked through the packing.

The doctor looked alarmed. "We'll check his blood. I have to determine if he needs a transfusion as well as identify the cause of this bleeding. It may just be a broken blood vessel. But it is important to make sure we are not missing something more serious."

Like their son, Atul's parents stayed silent. Worry shot through them. This ordeal was taking longer than expected, and they had left their other children alone to fend for themselves in a mud hut. What would become of them?

Four hours later, the doctor was reviewing the results of Atul's blood work. It was clear that the boy was anemic and required an urgent transfusion. The results of further tests, including a white blood cell count, platelets, INR, PTT and bleeding time all turned up normal.

But despite the blood transfusion, Atul showed no sign of improvement. Although the vomiting stopped, the child's nose just kept on bleeding. The boy remained in the pediatric ward for days, undergoing many more transfusions. But even with gastroenterology investigations, the source of the bleeding remained a medical mystery.

On the fifth day of Atul's hospital stay, the otolaryngologist, Dr. Malhotra, appeared. He conducted a quick exam, then took a cursory look inside the boy's mouth and nose. Satisfied that there was no active bleeding, the doctor grunted and left the room. In the hall, he scratched a few lines in Atul's chart and forgot about the little boy even before he returned his fountain pen to his jacket pocket.

After a week, the bleeding finally slowed to a crawl, and Atul, as listless and quiet as the day he arrived in hospital, was discharged without an explanation for the epistaxis. His discharge diagnosis read epistaxis NYD. In other words, the cause for it had not yet been determined.

Atul's worried parents bundled up their boy and carried him out of his room. As they passed the nursing station,

Atul let out a cough and a blast of blood shot from his nose. Without a sound, his mother pulled a tissue from her sack and wiped the blood, giving the gaggle of nurses sitting in their station a pleading stare.

The charge nurse had no choice. Sighing, she pointed to Atul's vacant hospital room, and the group turned and made its way back down the hall.

The doctor on duty was a plump fellow by the name of Dr. Baboo Tanoli. A pediatrician by training, he had graduated from the British system two decades earlier. Summoned by the charge nurse, the doctor arrived on the ward after lunch. He reviewed Atul's chart and entered the boy's room.

"Hello, little Atul," he said, smiling. "More bleeding, eh? Let's take a look."

With huge eyes, Atul gazed at the doctor.

Dr. Tanoli began his exam, paying particular attention to the boy's eyes. He was looking for signs of yellowing called sclera icterus. Next, he examined Atul's lungs and heart, liver and spleen. So far, he couldn't find a thing wrong with the child.

Using an otoscope, the doctor then peered into the cavern of Atul's nose. Blood dripped. Suddenly, Dr. Tanoli yelped and jumped back. He had seen something move up there, and one thing was for sure: it wasn't blood. He paged Dr. Malhotra, and described with excitement and fear the mobile mass he had seen in the patient's nostril.

An hour later, Dr. Malhotra was back in the ward. His white lab coat was flecked with food stains. His body smelled of spice and his breath was the only thing that had changed Atul's facial expression in weeks. As far as Atul was concerned, there was not much to like about the man. The doctor reached out and pushed back Atul's neck as if he were a doll. Then he looked up the boy's nose. Astonished, he confirmed there was indeed something in there that didn't belong. It was alive.

How could he have missed this during his previous exam? It must have been absent the first time around, he concluded, his hubris as impenetrable as ever. Well, at least he succeeded in the end. Grasping forceps, the doctor reached up the boy's nostril and captured the cause of Atul's misery: a seven-centimeter wriggling brown leech.

Within minutes, the bleeding slowed to a stop, and soon after, little Atul was released. He returned to his village more fearful of drinking water from the communal pond, which he now knew was home to leeches. He and his friends often played in the shallow water, and Atul had always loved dunking his head to see how long he could hold his breath. What he didn't know was that leeches will turn any accessible orifice into a home. By drinking and playing in the pond, Atul presented the unwelcome guest the perfect opportunity to swim up his nose and feed off his young food supply.

Leeches attach to their host by a sucker. They painlessly connect and suck blood using suction and by secreting mucus as well as the anticoagulant hirudin, which causes excessive bleeding. But leeches are not all bad. They are, in fact, so adept at improving blood flow that they are used in medical practice through a process called Hirudotherapy. After surgery, doctors attach leeches to the patient's wound to limit congestion of blood and improve healing. The little suckers have a field day then emerge as heroes. Fancy that.

TRACTOR ATTRACTION

40

John was a loner.

Raised on a 100-acre cattle farm in Oregon, he spent his early years home-schooled in a strict religious household. When he and his brother and sister had finished studying around the kitchen table, they got busy with chores. Life was harsh. Step out of line and you were standing in a corner, suffering the slap of Dad's belt across your bare hide.

On the first Monday of every month, John broke free of the farm. He accompanied his father to town on business, but while his dad spent the day attending meetings, John sat waiting for hours in the passenger seat of the truck, staring straight ahead.

At age nine, John discovered the glorious art of masturbation. With little other excitement in his life, he would pleasure himself in the privacy of a bedroom or bathroom four times a day.

One day, just as John was teetering on the verge of a dizzying explosion, his bedroom door swung open. His mother, carrying a basketful of freshly folded laundry, shrieked, as socks and underwear tumbled to the floor. Oddly excited by this sudden intrusion, John shot his load all over the bed. Shocked, wringing her hands on her apron, his mother turned and left, leaving the door, and John, gaping.

It took just seconds to zip his jeans. Then his father appeared in the doorway. His clothes splotched with grease and mud, he marched straight for John. Without a word, he grabbed his son by the ear and dragged him to the barn.

John knew what was coming. Despite himself, his fear mingled with excitement. He had been strapped and whipped many times before. Getting off on the familiar smell of manure and straw, John lay across the seat of a rusted old gas-powered backhoe tractor, and dropped his overalls and his underwear. He heard the leather belt swoosh from the loops of his father's pants and felt a tingle shoot through his legs. He focused on the ground, hiding his smile as his face turned red.

Each whip licked his skin harder than the last. The pain, so intense, was almost unbearable in its agony, shame and delight. It was a punishment John knew and longed for. When the thrashing stopped, his father stood straight. His breath came out ragged.

"That'll teach you," his father growled. "Now get up and check the herd."

John pulled up his pants and hobbled to the tractor. He

climbed up but squirmed when he tried to sit. With his flesh stinging, it would be a restless ride.

As John grew older, he would frequently steal out late at night, mount his beloved tractor and masturbate over the red rusted chassis like a rodeo cowboy on a bucking bull. He liked to leave his mark on its frame, a liquid tattoo of ownership. By age fifteen, he had christened her Deere, and in the privacy of his bedroom, penned her poems and love songs. Without friends, John obsessed about Deere, lovingly reciting her ballads in the flickering candlelight of the barn.

John's secret obsession permeated his life. His father beamed, manifested as a grunt and quick shake of his head, when John enrolled in a part-time mechanics program at a junior college. But the fact was, John's beloved tractor was at the center of nearly all of his conversations, at home and at school. His dorm room was adorned with photographs of himself and Deere in various poses throughout the farm.

"He's a total weirdo," his classmates agreed. And after a year in college, during which John was unable to establish even one friendship, he returned to the farm for the summer.

"I'm off to work on Deere," he called to his parents one summer evening after dinner. "She needs an oil change."

"You just changed it last week, what are they learnin' you at that school?" his father asked. Spawned from a line of farmers spanning generations, his dad was suspicious. He may not have earned a high school diploma but he knew more about the mechanics of farm work than his son could ever learn at college.

John ignored the question. He cleared his plate and set off

for the barn. John had loved his tractor every day since his return home and here he was, close to her again. John's dad heard the familiar roar of its motor, as he had dozens of times before.

The next morning at dawn, John's father headed to his son's room to wake him for the day's work, but John's bed lay made. Next, he checked the bathroom. No John. Expecting to find him frying eggs at the stove, he found, instead, a dark kitchen. Maybe he's already outside, his father thought.

As he approached the barn, he heard the idling engine. "You're up mighty early," John's father called, stepping inside. Then he froze. There was John, suspended by a safety harness wrapped around his neck. The other end was attached to the raised shovel of the tractor. One end of a long stick was taped to the control of the hydraulic lever of the backhoe shovel, while the other end was poised under his son's buttocks. In this contraption, pressure from his butt could raise or lower the lever. Raising the shovel caused it to rise, tightening the ligature around his neck.

An autopsy confirmed that John had died of asphyxiation. In an act of autoerotica, he had accidentally strangled himself.

Autoerotic behavior includes the act of masturbation coupled with near strangulation. It is classified as paraphilia (sexual deviation). The strangulation component — which may be accomplished by hanging (using various ligatures), immersion in water, self-strangulation, suffocation with bags, chest pressure, obstruction of the upper airway or other acts — results in hypoxia (low oxygen). Genital stimulation using hands is not always a component of autoerotica. The act is based on excitement arising from the danger of the practice, as well as the sensations associated with near strangulation during sexual gratification.

Accidental asphyxiation is more common than one might think. It has been bandied about as the possible cause of death in a number of famous people. Australian singer Michael Hutchence of the group INXS was found dead by a hotel maid in Room 524 of the Ritz-Carlton Hotel in Sydney, Australia. Some reports considered the cause of death to be autoerotic asphyxiation. Famous actor David Carradine hanged himself in a hotel room in Bangkok, Thailand, also reportedly due to autoerotic asphyxiation. A British member of parliament from Eastleigh, Stephen Milligan, was found dead in 1984. The scene revealed a wild combination of autoerotica, self-bondage and cross-dressing.

ENTRY WOUND

41

After three days of August heat, the stench drifted like smoke. It started as a sour odor tickling the nostrils of the occupants next to Apartment 321. But soon, it was everywhere, and all of the inhabitants on the third floor were pinching their noses. Finally, the superintendant rode the elevator up.

He knocked on the locked door, louder and longer with each unanswered rap. As if it had been left playing on repeat, Pink Floyd's *Dark Side of the Moon* was crooning from within, and man, did it stink. He should have grabbed his gas mask. Sighing, the super used his master key and then gagged as he pushed the door open.

Decay flew at him from every direction as he held his breath and headed to the bedroom, hunting for signs of life.

There it was, on the floor beside the bed. A rumpled, bloated corpse. There was only one name on this guy's lease: Ricardo.

Forensics sealed the room with requisite yellow tape and Detective Hardy entered the apartment wearing booties, gloves and a mask. Anne Spall, a technician who was similarly dressed, was already on the scene, clicking her camera. Waifish, she wore only black to match her shoulder length hair, and she had piercings, lots of them, dotting her face. She always looked like she took perverse pleasure in forensics work.

"I'm guessing suicide," Anne said, snapping away.

"What gave that away, the gun?" Hardy asked. He liked Anne, a bit too much for a man married only five years.

Ricardo had worked as a security guard at a mall. Now, lying on the floor, his head resting on a stained pillow, he wore only a white T-shirt. Buried beneath him was a Smith & Wesson sw1911 handgun, aluminum framed and alloyed with scandium in a black finish. The handgun contained a spent casing and five live rounds.

The detective noted that the body was in a mild state of decomposition and a major state of putrefaction. There was no obvious bullet entry site visible but Hardy was not in the mood to conduct a full exam of the decedent. He would gladly leave that work to the more well paid pathologists. He liked his job, probably even more than Anne liked hers. But let's face it, dead women were a lot more interesting than dead men.

Still, this one was no slouch. Items found at the scene included a wooden police baton, a tube of lubricating jelly, piles of well-thumbed pornographic magazines, a dozen empty beer bottles and a suicide note, written mainly in black ink with the final lines seemingly penned in blood. To make matters more interesting, a bloody pulp of tissue rested on top of the refrigerator in a mason jar filled with clear liquid. And photo albums containing unusual pictures were scattered around the room. Hardy completed his review and nodded to the attendants from the morgue.

Dressed in thin white disposable body suits, operating room caps and allergen free latex gloves, they tagged the body, zipped it into a standard body bag and carried the carcass on a gurney to the waiting van.

Ricardo's medical records disclosed a number of prior suicide attempts involving self-mutilation. A year ago, he had tried cutting off his penis requiring reversal by the skilled hands of the world-renowned urologist Dr. Norbert Ram.

Hardy had seen enough suicides that the details seemed irrelevant. It was suicide and that was that. Time to close the case and move on. He did, however, relish the opportunity to head down to Anne's office and review her photos from the scene.

The autopsy showed early signs of decomposition including bloating, discoloration and maggot infestation around body orifices. Both of Ricardo's wrists, as well as his nipples and the base of his penis, were scarred. One nipple was pierced as were his scrotum and penis. The other nipple was missing, having been freshly removed.

The pathologist, Dr. Packer, found no external evidence of an entry wound. Examination of the buttocks revealed a series of stellate tears radiating outward in a symmetrical starburst pattern. Unsure of the source of the pattern but suspicious nonetheless, the pathologist ordered an abdominal X-ray.

With a brow raised, the doctor looked at the image. On the abdominal films, he saw multiple radio-opaque objects of various shapes and sizes. There were cylinders and tubes throughout the large bowel that did not appear to have been swallowed. In the right chest, he noted the characteristic shape of a deformed cylindrical bullet.

Over the course of his career, Dr. Packer had seen many young dead men with bullets in their chests, but he had never seen an X-ray quite like this one. And where on earth was that mysterious gunshot wound? It was time to find out, he thought, as he gathered his bevy of scalpels and knives and began slicing up Ricardo.

It took a few minutes with both of his hands wrist-deep in Ricardo's pelvis and abdomen before Dr. Packer found the point of entry. There it was, right through the asshole.

The bullet had entered just proximal to the anus and had perforated the rectal mucosa. It tore through the sigmoid colon, ascending colon, right lobe of the liver, right hemi-diaphragm and middle lobe of the right lung before finally landing in the right pleural space. There was a half liter of blood there, and another liter had spilled into the abdominal cavity. Though the rectal mucosa was blackened, there was no actual gunshot residue evident.

The doctor found a half dozen objects inside Ricardo's rectum. Anything other than feces is an anal interloper, he thought. He pulled them out, one by one: gear shift knobs, a single lens from eyeglasses, an empty canister of whipped cream that thankfully had not been penetrated by the gunshot. Otherwise, this would have been an even messier business.

The autopsy concluded that Ricardo's death resulted from suicide carried out by an intra-rectal gunshot wound. Ricardo had not accidentally sat on the gun. He had, rather, pointed the barrel upward, then sat on top of it.

The tissue in the jar was a human nipple that had been used to write the bloody suicide note, like a pen dipped in ink. The photo albums depicted Ricardo engaged in various sexual acts with his wife. They were consistent with a history of sadomasochistic paraphilia.

Paraphilias are disorders where sexual arousal is sought from behavior that deviates from what is considered a normal range. More common in men, paraphilias include fetishism (arousal with inanimate objects), masochism (humiliation, beatings and/or torture), pedophilia (arousal from prepubescent children), frotteurism (rubbing against a person without consent) and transvestitism (cross-dressing, almost exclusively involving heterosexuals).

In this case, Ricardo exhibited evidence of both masochism and fetishism. His masochistic tendencies were obvious from the injuries to his penis and nipples while the objects inside his rectum represented his tendency toward fetishism. Likely feeling abandoned by his wife, who had recently left him and with whom he had shared his paraphilia, the terminal intra-rectal gunshot wound was meant to make a final statement.

Intra-rectal insertion of objects has been extensively reported in medical literature. Among many other items, a variety of bottles, fruits, vegetables, umbrellas and even a baseball and bat have been recorded to have found their way up the butt.

MODEL BEHAVIOR

42

After his wife left him for her personal trainer at the gym, Leslie moved to Concord, New Hampshire where life was slow and kind. He was past retirement and he'd had more than enough drama. It was time for some solitary living.

Leslie's favorite season, hands down, was fall. He loved the cool, comfortable temperatures and the lakes of golden leaves everywhere. So in September and October, he spent most weekends enjoying the long drive along the Kancamagus Scenic Byway through the middle of the White Mountains.

There was nothing lovelier than stopping at Franconia Notch State Park. Leslie pulled his Buick off Interstate 93 onto the gravel just outside the park and killed the ignition. With his packed lunch in hand, he trekked twenty minutes through the brush to a large clearing in the woods.

He was delighted to see a group of model airplane racers there. What a treat! Taking a seat on a knoll a hundred yards back, Leslie crossed his legs and watched the action from a distance.

Pylon racers are small radio-controlled propeller aircraft that shoot around pylons in a circular track at speeds of up to 150 miles per hour. Dependent on expert piloting, pylon racing is a hobby sport with pockets of enthusiasts across the country.

Harley flew a Snipp. With a fifty-one-inch wingspan and a Medusa brushless geared motor, it weighed just twenty-six ounces. Harley considered his plane a versatile, powerful, aerodynamic marvel. And he considered himself an awesome pilot. He often placed in the weekly races held in various cities in the New England states. As a result, his bedroom wall was lined with medal after medal.

For Harley, pylon racing was only a hobby, though. And as skilled as he was, he still wasn't competition for those who entered the National Championship Air Races. To complicate matters, despite Harley's love of racing miniature radio-controlled aircraft, his love of alcohol tended to compromise his judgment in the air. In fact, booze interfered with much more than his hobby. It affected pretty much every aspect of his life. Like Leslie, a man he had never met, Harley too had been abandoned by his wife. Now, his Snipp was all he had left to love.

On this particular fall day, Harley made it to the race just in time. But to his chagrin, he had left his flask of forty-proof whiskey sitting on the kitchen table back at his apartment.

It would be very hard to control the pylon racer while he was both bleary-eyed and in a state of alcohol withdrawal. Particularly if he got the shakes.

The drone of engines buzzed as a few spectators ringed the perimeter of the track. Harley steered his Snipp around the pylons but could not maintain his lead as his stomach contents refluxed into the back of his throat. He swallowed and tried to focus. As the nausea intensified, he slowed his aircraft in preparation for landing. His day was done. His heart wasn't in it. The fact was, Harley wanted a drink more than he wanted a model aircraft victory. And he knew it.

As Harley steered his plane to the ground, though, it suddenly veered left and came crashing down. To his horror, he watched his Snipp collide with someone sitting on a knoll overlooking the field. It was a remarkable stroke of bad luck. A clearing the size of two football fields, and some loser on a hill destroyed his baby!

At first, it seemed like a minor accident. The aircraft was small, after all. Harley and the few onlookers rushed to the man who was now lying flat. But as soon as Harley arrived on the scene, breathless, his face crimson, he realized he was in big trouble.

Leslie was disoriented. He had been sipping coffee from a thermos emblazoned with an American flag when the plane zoomed into view. It flew into the right upper quadrant of his abdomen then splintered into pieces. The pain flashed white. Leslie slumped over. Dizzy, he couldn't catch his breath. Before he passed out, the last image he saw was Harley, all 5 feet, 6 inches, 260 pounds of him, lumbering up the hill.

Harley dialed an ambulance after seeing that the man on the ground was not moving a muscle. He looked like he was sleeping, but when Harley pushed him over onto his back, he found that the man was no longer breathing.

"Is there a doctor here?" Harley shouted to the group of shocked onlookers.

The wife of another flier rushed to Leslie. She was a nurse. She tried, unsuccessfully, to locate a pulse in Leslie's wrist and neck. But she was skittish about initiating CPR. So she stood with the others and watched the man die.

The ambulance arrived a full twenty-six minutes after the call.

"He's dead," said the medic. "What happened?"

Harley was terrified. He couldn't speak. Did he really just kill someone with his Snipp?

"This guy lost control of his plane," exclaimed another flier, pointing at Harley then turning to the man on the grass. "And it crashed into that guy."

The medics found little external evidence of trauma. It just wasn't clear what had killed Leslie. Unsure if they were standing in the middle of a crime scene, the medics waited for police to arrive before wrapping the body and carting it to the morgue for an autopsy. They wondered about the cause of death, though, and asked the morgue attendant to give them a call when there was an answer.

The pathologist on duty, Dr. Levi Dillon, was new on the job. He had just finished four years of postgraduate training in pathology. An electric man with a magnetic personality, Levi was known for his endless energy.

He slit Leslie's abdomen. Inside, he found liters of clotted and fresh blood. The source of bleeding was immediately apparent. Leslie's liver had been snipped in half by the impact of a model aircraft traveling at about 100 miles per hour.

As rare as it is to die in an airplane crash, the likelihood of dying from one while firmly planted on the ground is remarkably small. And the chance of meeting your death from a crash involving a craft weighing just over two pounds is too small to calculate. Especially when the driver, like Harley, was dead sober.

BREATHE EASY

43

For as long as she could remember, Emma had been known as a sneezer and wheezer. In fact, her earliest memories were of car rides to the emergency department where she was gasping for breath in the back seat. At the hospital, she would lie under a cool moist tent and feel mentholated aerosolized droplets being pumped inside.

Her asthma attacks came with little warning. There were so many seemingly innocent precipitants: a cold virus, pollen, too much exertion. It seemed as though everyday life could prompt a life-threatening episode. As a result, Emma lived a sheltered existence. She had few friends.

When Emma was six, her family moved from the suburbs to an apartment downtown, just one block from a hospital. She hated the sight of concrete sidewalks and the shriek of sirens outside her bedroom window but living so close to medical help brought her parents great comfort.

Whereas many kids experience less frequent and intense asthma episodes as they age, Emma's condition grew worse through her teens and early twenties. By the time she turned thirty-two, she had taken so many courses of prednisone that she had become osteopenic. Bone density studies showed that she had the skeletal strength of a woman twice her age. Now Emma worried about broken hips and arthritic knees.

Prednisone, a synthetic steroid, is a wonder drug that hit the market in the 1960s and is an example of a classic double-edged medical sword. It is a powerful anti-inflammatory medicine that can resolve all manner of diseases with tantalizing speed. As a result, the patient is often left with delusions of being cured.

In reality, however, prolonged chronic use and at times even brief courses of the drug can wreak havoc on the body's ability to fight infection. On one hand, prednisone can create as many problems as it fixes, including mood swings, psychosis, hypertension, diabetes and a host of other conditions. But on the other hand, in many cases, it is the best that medicine can offer for bringing patients relief.

Emma was used to one and two week treatments of prednisone in tapering doses to quiet her asthma episodes. At times, her wheezing and shortness of breath became so severe that she faced the terror of impending death, only to click back to normal after a large intravenous dose of the miracle drug. Usually, though, all she needed was a simple spray from her collection of inhalers to normalize her ragged breathing.

So far, she had yet to stab herself in the thigh with her EpiPen but it was never far from her hand.

Friday began like any other day. Emma showered and dressed. She walked the ten minutes to the bus stop and caught the 8:15 bus. A half hour ride into the city would leave her fifteen minutes for a coffee before she took her cubicle at the call center. She hated public transport. She was punctual by nature but buses were never on time and to make matters worse, the drivers never smiled. Annoyed to be ten minutes late, she rushed into the building only to find the elevator out of service — again.

Her supervisor would be furious. She was a squat woman the same age as Emma, and it was clear that she enjoyed picking on a select club of employees. Emma was at the top of her hate list.

Hurrying up the five flights of stairs, Emma had to stop halfway. She was breathing hard. She needed a quick fix. At the third floor, she rested against the wall and pulled her blue inhaler from her purse. She pushed its top and sucked the cool mist deep into her airways. After decades of practice, Emma was expert at maximizing the effect of the drug with a perfectly choreographed spray and intake of breath. She was like a sadly addicted smoker. She took the last two flights slowly, and when she reached the top, she bent over, hands on knees, to breathe. Not surprisingly, her supervisor was unsympathetic.

"Are you working or choking today?" the bitch barked.

Unable to complete a full sentence, Emma stood, walked to her desk, and sprayed her throat a few more times with each inhaler in her collection. One of them had to work. Her supervisor hovered over her desk, arms crossed.

"If you can't arrive on time and do your job without rasping into the phone, then I suggest you quit," she said.

Emma could feel the wheezing slow. She rummaged through her purse for the prednisone she had just picked up at the pharmacy near her new physician's office.

Emma's GP had retired six months ago. Although no family doctors in her area were accepting new patients, Emma had been lucky. When her retiring GP put in a word for her, his colleague agreed to take her on.

The verdict was still out on the new doctor. Emma saw right away that the man was too old. Plus, his office was a mess. If he wasn't concerned enough to keep his belongings in order, how in the world could his patients trust the man to look after their ailments? Emma looked at the pills she had spilled into her hand. They looked different. Her usual prednisone pills were round and white, scored down the center. These were round and scored, yes, but they were beige.

Under the bitch's watchful eye, Emma popped two 10 milligram tablets, donned her headset, and pressed a button. Ten minutes later, she was in the midst of her third call.

"OTT Contact Industries, how may I help you?" Emma said. Her voice was sweet but hoarse.

As the conversation continued, Emma felt a rising panic in her throat. Her breaths came out fast and her chest felt like it was shrinking. Soon, she was gasping. Unable to draw air, she clutched her throat. Before passing out, she looked up to see her supervisor standing over her, her mouth in the shape of the letter O.

The bum elevator delayed the medics, who, like Emma, had to climb the stairs. As fast as possible, they stuck a tube down her throat but her airways were so tight that they could not manually ventilate her. The epinephrine squirted directly into her lungs had no effect. Emma descended into ventricular fibrillation. Her heart, unable to rhythmically contract, quivered like Jell-O.

The postmortem examination showed findings of an acute asthma attack. Tenacious casts of mucus had occluded Emma's airways, making it impossible for her to breathe. Her bronchial vessels were congested and edematous and the bronchial smooth muscle layer was enlarged.

Had she cut corners, the pathologist, Dr. Grosse, would have chalked up this case to another sudden death from asthma. But she was a sweep-every-corner woman. So she got to work reviewing the police notes from their interview with the supervisor at the call center where Emma died. The woman had explained that Emma collapsed about fifteen minutes after taking a few pills from a bottle in her purse.

As all of Emma's belongings had been transported with her corpse to the coroner's office, Dr. Grosse took the opportunity to examine their contents. She unzipped the purse and after sifting through the half dozen inhalers and an EpiPen, she was startled to discover a single pill bottle, nearly full, containing a prescription for 40 milligram tablets of propranolol.

Developed by Scottish physician James W. Black, propranolol

was the first beta-blocker ever synthesized. A breakthrough in the treatment of high blood pressure and heart attacks, the drug was the world's bestseller at the time of its development, a title it held until the introduction of cimetidine, an anti-ulcer medication. Remarkably, Dr. Black, who went on to win a Nobel Prize in medicine in 1988, also synthesized cimetidine. He died in 2010.

Dr. Grosse shook her head. Why would a woman with a lifelong history of asthma swallow propranolol during an asthma attack? There is only one condition in which a beta-blocker can never be used, and that condition is asthma. That's because propranolol worsens asthma by constricting airways and blocking the effects of the medications found in inhalers.

Beck's Pharmacy was located on the southeast corner of Park and Woodbine in Chicago on the ground floor of a ten-story commercial building. The pharmacist who ran the place was startled to receive a call from the coroner who explained that an investigation into the recent death of a patient was underway. Dr. Grosse was careful not to mention Emma's name just in case the pharmacy records, which would soon be impounded under a court order, then mysteriously vanished.

The old pharmacist was worried. He had no idea who the dead patient might be. He felt helpless as he hung up the phone, wishing he had retired like his wife had been nagging him to do for years.

When the police arrived with the order, the pharmacist took his time leafing through prescriptions. With a hand shaky from fear and Parkinson's, he found the single script in Emma's name.

In this case, there was no lockbox of documents. Dr. Grosse simply needed to know who wrote the prescription for propranolol. Even medical students knew the importance of asking a patient about asthma before handing over a prescription.

What Dr. Grosse discovered was not entirely unexpected. The script, though bordering on illegible, was for prednisone, not propranolol. Instead of verifying the handwriting, the pharmacist had taken his best guess. In the end, Emma's sudden death from asthma was the result of the domino effect. A series of errors began with a doctor's poor penmanship followed by the fact that an old pharmacist needed new glasses, and ended with a trusting patient who didn't stop to read the label on the bottle of pills she relied on to save her life.

ANY WAY YOU SLICE IT

44

"Live once and live well." That was Gil's motto whether that meant stripping down to his shorts to hit the beach or licking his fingers after enjoying a sumptuous feast. The bottom line was, Gil would do pretty much anything to boost his sexual arousal. Gil was into innocent exploration, testing new ways to make himself shoot his load. But when he stumbled upon the pleasure of strangling his penis, he was ecstatic.

He came upon it by chance. A dozen years ago, he was a typical twenty-four-year-old getting off on porn flicks when he found himself mesmerized by a particular blond actor who resembled Fabio. Gil watched in amazement as the man's partner placed rubber rings around both men's erect members, and bang! They both stayed happily hard for the next hour of fun.

Gil didn't understand the mechanics. In fact, a ring around the penis occludes blood flow after an erection, forcing the blood to stay put inside the engorged penis. All Gil cared about was heading pronto to the hardware store for some rings, large nuts, and rubber bands.

It was time for some serious experimentation. Quickly, elastic bands shot to the top of Gil's Favorite Toy List. Because they are more expandable depending on how many times they are looped, the elastics were the ultimate in hedonism. Gil could manipulate one to provide the ultimate in personal satisfaction.

One Saturday evening at home, Gil smoked a joint and as usual, the drug made him horny. He flicked on his favorite porn flick and sat for hours, watching and rubbing until his shoulder ached and the skin on his penis became chafed. Then, spying an empty Gatorade bottle beside the TV, he felt a new thought forming in his mind, something unique, never seen before.

Clutching the plastic bottle by the neck, he removed the top, forced his penis into its mouth and continued his masturbation marathon. Sensations raged through his loins. He was building toward one great moment, he thought, letting his member swell with pride and joy. That is, until thirty minutes later, when his shoulder became so sore it was time to stop, and he tried to withdraw himself from the bottle's jaws.

Through the plastic, Gil's penis resembled the trunk of a baby elephant. It was painfully clear that the blood could not escape the tight grip of the bottleneck. For a long time, men have been accused of thinking with their little heads. But now, Gil's little head was strangled.

With sweat sliding shamefully down his forehead, Gil tugged until finally it dawned on him that this problem was big. Too big. His mind whirred into overdrive. How many vice presidents of commercial banks head to the hospital with their penis in a bottle? How would he explain himself? Perhaps he could say he had been held captive by a violent band of homosexual recyclers. Or that he had awoken with a hard-on and needed to relieve himself in the toilet only to fall directly into an open bottle lying on the carpet. Could he claim his penis felt thirsty?

Any way you sliced it, if word got out that Gil had an incarcerated penis, it could mean a life of unemployment. Even in a city of a million people, news like this travels.

The solution seemed obvious. A steak knife. Holding the bottle in place, Gil shuffled to the kitchen and went to work. He opened a drawer and pulled out the tool. Then he started sawing the plastic bottle. In the meantime, as the effects of the marijuana waned, the pain soared.

Gil was at a disadvantage. He had to be careful. He couldn't merely hack away. If his hand slipped, the stakes were high. At the same time, the elephant trunk that his penis had morphed into just kept growing until it was engorged and edematous. Its sides were squashed against the half-liter bottle. It was barely contained.

Looking like a circus freak in a pelvic sideshow, Gil panicked. Worst of all, he had to pee. What now? Hadn't he read somewhere that long parts of the body would be okay even without blood flow? Unlike the kidneys, lungs and liver, the penis wasn't considered a transplantable organ. But in the very worst case scenario, could the penis survive on ice in a cooler — temporarily separated from its blood supply?

Gil couldn't think straight. All he knew was if he didn't get that bottle off soon, he would spend his miserable life peeing out of a hole the size of his belly button. In agony, he tried to pull up his pants but there was no way. But there was also no way he could walk down the streets of downtown with a bottle sticking out of his open fly.

There was nothing left to do. Gil found the phone and called an ambulance. He could transfer to another branch of the bank in another city far, far away. At the hospital, he would have to remember not to allow photographs. He would refuse to sign a waiver.

The paramedics were dumbfounded by what was inside Gil's apartment. Not one of them had ever seen what appeared to be a case of penile strangulation. The two ambulance attendants were bug-eyed and silent. Besides cracking a joke or busting into hysterics, what was there to say? They lifted Gil onto a stretcher and as he and the bottle lay pointing upward, they ferried him to hospital.

The emergency department was as loud as a factory floor. As soon as Gil was transferred into the resuscitation room, however, the noise suddenly ceased.

The physician was at a loss. Whom should she call? A urologist? An orthopedic surgeon? A handyman or engineer? She set up an IV and considered suprapubic catheterization just in case Gil's bladder was in danger of bursting. Then she summoned a urologist, orthopedic surgeon, hospital handyman and engineer. She needed all the help she could get.

The crack team examined Gil. By then, he was so doped up on intravenous Valium that he couldn't care less if they pickled his penis and testicles and replaced them with a vagina and ovaries.

Plans were drawn, diagrams and sketches were proposed. Finally, after four long minutes of intense decision making, with each member of the dream team jostling for a say, it was decided that the bottle would be cut using an iron saw. Soon, the room was all zigs and zags, with each team member taking a turn with the device, the nurses mopping sweat from the brows of the doctors and tradesmen.

After a twenty-minute struggle involving the saw followed by forceps, a long swollen object looking too much like a shar-pei dog was born and the entire room seemed to sigh. Because the swelling prevented Gil from peeing, a catheter, inserted into the shaft of his member, drained the night's urine. After a full week of hospitalization, Gil and his penis were finally free.

Having called in sick to work citing a medical emergency, Gil spent the next week recuperating in bed. He told the powers that be at his company that he had undergone an appendectomy and that the surgery had been complicated by an infection. As far he knew, no one was the wiser but he was careful never to step foot inside that hospital again.

Penile strangulation has rarely been reported in literature. In 1999, separate grades of penile injury were devised to help define the term. The first, Grade I, results in edema of the distal portion of the penis without skin or urethral injury. The grading ascends all the way up to Grade V, which leaves the sufferer with gangrene, necrosis or complete amputation of the member. In one case report, a victim too embarrassed to seek help, stayed put at home for nearly two weeks. That unwise decision resulted in penile necrosis, bilateral kidney infections, pneumonia and finally, death.

TRICK OR TREAT

45

Shortly after his father abandoned him, Anton decided to commit murder. His dad was slime. He had been caught in bed with the daughter of a close friend, and split for Poland, just like that. He was a rich man, but after a few months, stopped sending money to his family at home. So Anton was forced to drop out of medical school to support his mother and sister. At night, he spent hours surfing the internet, fantasizing about how his father would die.

Even before his dad left, there was nothing normal about Anton. He was a perennially unpopular boy who could not seem to form friendships. Growing up, he had never kissed a girl. As an adult, his occasional experiments with cheap prostitutes left him feeling like a loser.

Anton earned a living stocking shelves at the local

supermarket but when he lost his job due to antisocial behavior, he pooled all of his money and bought a one-way ticket to Poland. He found his father, who was living with his granddad, in a small town called Chelersk. After the reunion, Anton moved in. Months passed. Although Anton's hatred of his father seethed, he was adept at hiding it. He was preoccupied with his plan to trap and kill the old asshole. But he had to humiliate him first.

It took days to prepare the basement, an area of the home his father seemed to avoid. Anton spread out a large sheet of waterproof polyurethane tarp, positioned a heavy chain with a hook over a wooden support in the unfinished ceiling and arranged the tools he had brought from home. The screwdriver was his prime weapon.

It was harder than expected to lure his father downstairs. Cajoling would seem suspicious so he gave up mentioning the basement when his father didn't bite. The following day, it rained hard, giving Anton a stroke of genius.

In the study, he found his father sitting in a wingback leather chair, his legs stretched on an ottoman. He was immersed in a newspaper.

"Father," Anton said. "It looks as though the basement is leaking from the rain. What would you like me to do?"

Disgusted, as he always seemed to be, his father rose, and marched to the stairs, with Anton trailing behind him. As his father took the first step down, Anton gave him a two-handed shove. He watched the man topple down the steep stairs and hit the floor with a slam.

Groaning and dazed, his left hip fractured, Anton's father

opened his eyes just in time to see the screwdriver plunge into his chest, again and again and again. The sharp tool punctured his chest wall, repeatedly stabbing his heart. Anton watched his father's expression turn from shock to fear to dread in the seconds it took him to die.

The event, however, had not gone entirely according to plan. Anton had hoped that his father would land on top of the tarp but he had fallen short. Now, Anton had to drag a 250-pound corpse across the basement floor, leaving a wide bloody trail.

Anton was soaking through his shirt. Now came the hard part, the best part, the climax of the show. Fastening the chain and hook around his father's legs, he began hoisting the corpse until it was suspended over the wooden beam like the carcass of a cow in an abattoir.

That's when Anton decapitated the man whose genes he shared. He used a military knife he had bought months back, just for this purpose, and sawed his father's neck. After wiping his own face of sweat and blood, he grabbed the freed head by its hair and ascended the staircase where just minutes before, his father had tumbled in the opposite direction.

Anton and his father's head spent the rest of the evening alone, in the privacy of Anton's bedroom. Now it was Anton's turn to take control. For eight hours straight, he painstakingly removed the scalp and face from his father's cranium. At five the next morning, he looked at his handiwork and smiled. Then came the fun part. Anton returned to the top of the stairs, kicked the head like a soccer ball into the basement and turned back to the kitchen before it came to rest.

"Thanks, Dad," Anton thought. His medical school training, however briefly his father had paid for it, had served him well. And now he would prove it. Using thick 1-0 sutures, he sewed up the bloody scalp and face. Having created a real-life mask, he carefully dried it with salt to prevent decomposition.

That afternoon, Anton, gripped by psychosis, shaved his own head and using double-sided carpet tape, he pulled the mask over it. He made his way to his father's closet and chose an outfit to wear, completing it with a hat, scarf and glasses. Then, dressed as his dad from hair to toe, he strolled through town.

Seated on a park bench, Anton saw his grandfather walk by. He motioned him to the bench and the two conversed. His grandfather had no idea that he was talking to his grandson wearing the scalp and face of his own son. Returning home, the two men shared eggs and toast, reminiscing about the past.

After a few more hours together, though, Anton's grandfather felt an itch of suspicion. His son's voice seemed higher, and despite the old man's fading eyesight, he sensed something was wrong. He searched the house, and when he found a headless corpse in the basement, suspended upside down by chains from a supporting girder, he nearly fainted. But not before he called the police.

Anton was suspicious, too. His granddad had been squinting at him and kept making excuses to leave the room. When he heard the sound of the phone being dialed, he knew it was only a matter of time. He could kill his grandfather too, of course, but as fear shot through his loins, all Anton could do was fling open the front door, race across the street, and hide behind the fat trunk of a tree. From there, he heard a siren wail closer, then he watched as cops banged on the front door of the house.

Anton stayed hidden for the night. But the next day, when he returned to the park bench, still wearing his macabre mask, the police were there, waiting. When a crime is so heinous that it defies belief, it is almost always perpetrated by a person with extreme mental illness. This murder-decapitation-scalping-mask case is the only published one of its kind. Clearly, the killer was living deep in psychosis.

Psychosis renders the sufferer out of touch with reality. Characterized by false beliefs (delusions), and visual or auditory hallucinations, psychosis is a fundamental feature of schizophrenia. Psychosis may also be caused by alcohol, illegal drugs, dementia, steroids and infections, to name only a few. And yet as debilitating as psychosis can be, patients who suffer with it do not tend to decapitate a person, let alone create and wear a mask of human flesh.

BROKEN HEARTED

46

Brigitte was surprised to find that college life was quiet. Always studious, she had expected more from her first month of classes. Too fast, she was becoming one of those bored freshmen who scribbled notes then retired to a library cubicle until her lids dropped.

Upon arriving at school, Brigitte had moved into a small off-campus apartment, sight unseen. It turned out to be a ground floor two-bedroom with a porch leading to the back-yard. While she loved being able to head out to the lovely garden, Brigitte was concerned about the easy access to the apartment through the back. Like her parents did at home, she would have to affix security tape to the sliding glass door, which would make it harder to shatter with a bat or stick. Still, if someone was intent on breaking the glass, Brigitte knew there was little she could do to stop him, aside from installing a costly alarm system.

Like Brigitte, her roommates, Nibaal and Cassie, were hoping to get into graduate school after college. The trio made a pact. They would hit the books and churn out 4.0 grade point averages. No late night partying for them.

One night, after studying for hours, Brigitte and her friends took a break. Cassie dropped iced cubes and a paper umbrella into each girl's tea and the three friends sat around the table clinking glasses. It had been a productive night. The girls sipped their drinks as the conversation turned to their meager social lives.

"I've never even sipped an alcoholic drink," said Cassie by way of explaining why parties weren't her thing.

"Me neither," Nibaal agreed. "My parents would kill me if they caught me drinking. That's literal, not figurative. I mean they would actually stone me to death. They're a bit fanatical."

Wow, Brigitte thought. She could understand abstinence from drugs. She herself had never even seen a joint. But alcohol was ubiquitous on campus. It was hard to imagine, but maybe her friends' childhoods had been even more rigid than her own.

"You're not missing much," Brigitte said. "Eventually, alcohol makes your head or your stomach ache, or both."

Still, Brigitte did enjoy the odd cocktail. And drinking with friends would be fun. She needed some fun about now. The worst they could say was no.

"Would you guys ever think of maybe having cocktails one night if it were just us three? I mean, it would be safer than being at some bar, and we'd have fun together," Brigitte said.

"I guess so," Nibaal said, a smile pulling at her mouth. "As long as there's no chance my parents or brothers could ever find out." Her smile faded. "If I was caught drunk, you two would have one less person to compete with for a graduate school position."

A week later, Brigitte stepped into a liquor store for the first time. She passed by the selection of beers lining the shallow fridge across the wall and headed straight for the wine racks. Satisfied that no bottle cost more than ten dollars, she placed them all in a box, paid, and carried her cargo to the back seat of her Smart car. At home, she stowed the contraband in the fridge, then checked the cleaning schedule. It was her turn to tackle the kitchen, so she wiped counters and sprayed windows until they were so clean she could barely see them.

The three girls made a new pact. They would study until early evening. At nine o'clock, their first party would begin. For four hours straight, they crammed for their economics and marketing exams. When the alarm buzzed at 9 p.m., they closed their books and set aside their notes. Brigitte put on a Scissor Sisters CD and twisted open a bottle of Smoking Loon Syrah 2007.

The girls took turns pouring the wine into long-stemmed glasses. After downing the first bottle, split evenly, they all started to shed their inhibitions. Cassie was the first to feel its effects as she stumbled from euphoria to nausea. Her slurred speech made it hard for the girls to understand her.

Nibaal wondered why she had waited so long to try this fantastic concoction, forgetting for the hazy moment that doing so was punishable by death in her family. She made a mental note to change her name to Mary White and walk away from her past for good. As if.

Brigitte was ecstatic. She had been fantasizing about her roommates for too long. It had started the first time she had opened the bathroom door while Nibaal was showering. Now she entered unannounced all the time, feigning surprise that the room was occupied. She used every opportunity to glimpse the girls in their underwear, or if she was lucky, completely undressed. Oh, how she would love to get her roommates naked in bed, or on the couch or on the carpet or in the kitchen or on a chair. It didn't matter to her. As long as their bare skin could touch.

As it turned out, Brigitte had a much deeper history of alcohol use than she had let on. Twisting open the second bottle, she was feeling emboldened by the wine's effects and made her way to the middle of the room. Swaying to the rhythm of *Ta-Dah*, Brigitte grabbed hold of Nibaal's wrist and pulled her close. As Brigitte and Nibaal danced, ever closer, touching each other's arms and necks, all Cassie could think of was the toilet. She raced toward it, dropped down on the porcelain tiles and vomited the undigested lasagna dinner she had enjoyed only an hour before.

Nibaal languished in the attention up and down her body. It all felt so new. Besides alcohol, there were so many things she hadn't tried. But although Brigitte's caresses were soft and warm, something definitely felt wrong. Nibaal was heterosexual. So when Brigitte's mouth tried to find hers, she felt her face turning away.

The humiliation of rejection was fueled by the wine, and

Brigitte had to escape. How could she ever face her room-mates again? Running, she headed straight for the back porch — straight through the spotless glass door. Hundreds of shards of glass shattered like flying diamonds onto the concrete and Brigitte, shocked by the sudden smash, fell forward.

The noise was brief but loud. As Cassie snoozed on the toilet seat, vomit still spooling from her mouth, Brigitte lay motionless. Nibaal ran to her side. There was no blood on the scene, no lacerated artery, no head injury. Just glass, lots and lots of glass, twinkling.

By the time the police arrived, Nibaal was hysterical. As soon as her parents found out that Brigitte was dead, Nibaal knew she would be joining her friend. Her days on earth were numbered.

Brigitte's corpse was transferred to the coroner's office where it remained refrigerated until Monday morning. The autopsy revealed that liters of clotted blood had lodged in her thorax.

The coroner found a triangular glass shard, the size of a small knife, deeply embedded in the left ventricle of Brigitte's heart. She had run through the window alive but had fallen on the shard as if it had been the point of a sword. It had penetrated her left chest wall, between the fifth and sixth ribs, and pierced the apex of her left ventricle at a forty degree angle. Brigitte had exsanguinated through a stab wound into her chest.

When they heard what happened, Nibaal's parents could not believe their daughter had acted so irresponsibly. They allowed her to continue breathing, however, and to continue her studies, as long as she swore off alcohol forever. Cassie had a harder time dealing with Brigitte's sudden death. Unable to concentrate on her studies, she dropped out of college. And to numb the pain of the horrible memory, she took up drinking. Lots. Any alcohol she could get her pretty little hands on.

GOSSYPIBOMA

47

Reggie had expected improvement by now. Apparently, the surgery had gone smoothly and every day he was supposed to feel better. But here he was, hacking his lungs out every morning, afternoon and evening.

He knew his prognosis was excellent. Not only had the doctor told him so, but Reggie had taken the time to Google "papillary thyroid cancer" and he had even reviewed his own medical chart. Still, he looked forward to hearing the good news from his surgeon.

Reggie had figured that the procedure was going to cause some discomfort. Let's face it, they were slitting open his neck. He also knew that given the risks of papillary thyroid cancer, he would be damn lucky if it hadn't spread.

At the same time, though, he had initial misgivings about

Dr. Sheppard's ability to perform the neck dissection. The guy was — in a word — old. He repeated questions he already had the answer to, and the tremor in his hands was a bad start. Right about now, Reggie was thanking God that his eyes had opened after the operation. Dr. Sheppard looked at the dressing covering the patient's neck.

"We caught it early," the doctor said to Reggie. "You were lucky. Your GP did a good job identifying the mass in the first place. A lot of doctors would have missed this until it was too late."

Dr. Sheppard peeled back the protective Steri-Strips, exposing the wound for the first time in a week. Squinting at the incision over the top of his glasses, the doctor was pleased to see a thin pink line running across the bottom of Reggie's neck. Clean and smooth, the scar showed no evidence of infection, swelling or bleeding. The doctor placed a small bandage over the wound.

Taking a seat behind his desk, he opened the manila folder in front of him and flipped through the pages inside, searching for the operative report. Although Dr. Sheppard had performed the surgery only a week back, he scratched his head. He could not recall anything about the operation. It was frightening, these gaps in his memory. They were growing. The doctor could barely recognize the patient facing him.

In his long career, Dr. Sheppard had operated on hundreds of thyroid glands. Had this particular thyroidectomy been challenging? As much as he tried to concentrate on last week's events, he found they had been washed away, as if by a tide. He could catch only snippets of scenes. He remembered, for instance, making the decision to arrange a complete, rather than partial, thyroidectomy for the young man.

He reviewed the notes in the patient's chart. After the initial biopsy of the neck mass had come back positive for papillary carcinoma, the doctor had determined that removing the entire thyroid would give Reggie the best chance of survival. He had faced a few problems. The inferior thyroid artery turned out to be larger than he had expected. There may have been some difficulties with the simple act of parathyroid autotransplantation. He couldn't remember. There had been a lot more bleeding than usual too, but nothing that he hadn't been able to tackle with a few sponges.

Minutes dragged on. The doctor read through the chart, struggling to call up details. All the while, Reggie hacked and coughed into tissues.

Frustrated with his fading memory, the doctor looked at his patient. I'm in my early seventies, Dr. Sheppard thought. It's time to hang up my scalpel, he decided, hoping that he would remember this epiphany tomorrow. He looked down at the chart again. At least he could still understand what he was reading.

"So, Reggie," the doctor said. "The pathology report says that the resection margins were clear of tumor. The neck dissection was clear. Lymph nodes were clear. There's no indication the cancer has spread. I'll leave the final say to the oncologist, but I'm very pleased with the result." Dr. Sheppard's monologue was punctuated by coughing and wheezes from his patient. "Don't worry," the doctor added. "Coughing after this procedure is common."

Reggie was excited by the news. But the fact was, he felt dreadfully sick. His neck was still sore and the persistent feather tickling the back of his throat was driving him mad. Not only was he constantly interrupting himself with his own coughing fits, but even the doctor had trouble finishing a sentence with all of his hacking.

"Coughing is common in the first few days following this procedure," Dr. Sheppard said again, as if he were reassuring himself. He went on. "Your throat is probably sore from the endotracheal tube. Give it a few days and it will improve. If you're still troubled over the weekend, call the office. I can always take a look with a scope."

Reggie shook hands with the good doctor and left the office. Down the street, he hopped on the subway. After only two stations, the car stopped mid-tunnel. No announcement, nothing. Public transport sucked. What was so attractive about taking three times as long to get somewhere? In the humid semidarkness, the minutes stretched. Reggie began to feel his throat tighten. What the heck? Was this anxiety? A complication? Heat stroke?

Reggie started to shake as claustrophobia sealed him in. He wiped his sweaty forehead and coughed again and again into his sleeve. His throat felt raw. The walls seemed to be creeping closer from all sides. Passengers, assuming Reggie was infected with a virus they could catch, stepped back inches at a time until he was loosely surrounded by a small circle of backs.

After nearly fifteen minutes, the subway squealed and lurched forward. Just the movement alone, knowing he was going home, made Reggie feel better. By the time he reached his stop though, he was seeing stars. He stood up, immersed in doom. His neck felt as if it might snap. What if he was dying? The thought forced his feet forward, and he stepped out of the subway into the light.

After 100 yards, Reggie stopped to catch his breath by leaning on the trunk of an enormous tree. He gasped and coughed. He hugged the tree for help. Something was stuck in his throat and he was suffocating. He reached for his cell phone and hit the first number on his speed dial before flopping to the ground.

Fellow pedestrians flocked to the side of the man lying blue-faced on the grass, his eyes open and bloodshot. Minutes later, an ambulance arrived but it was a basic responder unit, unable to do more than simple CPR. As a result, Reggie was dead before reaching the hospital. In the emergency room, the emergency had already passed. There was nothing left to do.

The pathologist presumed that the man had died from a pulmonary embolism. It was a feared postoperative complication in cancer patients. After lying immobile for so long after an operation, blood clots form in the patient's leg veins. The blood pulls away from its site of origin, and embolizes, traveling through the venous system into the right side of the heart before lodging in the blood vessels of the lungs. The larger the clot, the more likely the patient will die from it.

But here, there was another explanation.

"Well, I'll be," mumbled the pathologist to no one in particular as he fished inside Reggie's neck. He had used an incision perpendicular to, but larger than, the careful line created by Dr. Sheppard. The pathologist didn't need to be so careful. At this point, he could saw his way in.

Looking through the gaping wound into the trachea, he found the culprit. It had been there all the time. A gossypiboma.

The surgeon and operating room staff had miscounted when they were cleaning up after the operation. Inside Reggie's neck, they had left behind a sponge. Over the course of a week, the sponge had gradually migrated from the wound inwards, before erupting into the trachea and blocking Reggie's airway like a beaver dam.

Gossypibomas are more common in intra-abdominal surgeries where they cause infections and persistent pain. A sponge left near an airway is rarer and more lethal.

The next day, Dr. Sheppard opened his door to a knock. There, standing before him, was an agent of the hospital's Medical Review Board and, just as the doctor had prophesied, it was time to hung up his scalpel for good. But when he was questioned about his fatal error, a funny thing happened. Dr. Sheppard couldn't recall the case.

NAMED

48

The police car rolled down the quiet residential street, passing manicured lawns, until it reached the address in the middle class suburb. The phone call had come into the station just a half hour ago. It was a concerned neighbor reporting that she had heard a loud fight. There had been screaming and sounds of breaking glass, she said. So she had waited until everything went quiet, then picked up the phone.

The front steps were marked with bloody footprints. The door was ajar. Sergeant Anderson used the muzzle of his Kimber M1911A1 pistol to push it open. Leading his partner, Anderson crept forward. Pointing their guns, the two cops advanced a few feet beyond the foyer. Anderson moved down the hall toward the kitchen, following the footprints.

"Police Department!" he shouted. "Identify yourself!"

Then he saw it. A puddle of blood in the hallway. It was running like a slow creek from the dining room where the sergeant found the body lying prone, arms tucked beneath his torso. The man was covered in so much blood, he looked like he had on Santa's suit.

"Send Homicide," Anderson said in a dead voice into his radio before he and his partner began scouring the house for occupants. Room to room they went, pulling open closet doors, peeking under beds. After the search, the all-clear was sounded. There were no further bodies, dead or alive, in this house.

Within minutes, police swarmed the home. Wearing blue jackets with HOMICIDE blazing across the back in bright yellow letters, a blend of technicians and detectives went about their business. They photographed the scene from dozens of angles then began hunting for clues. The dining room was cluttered and chaotic, with overturned lamps and chairs, and cracked mirror slices on the floor. The walls were bloody.

Detective Browning was on the case. He learned that the corpse belonged to Hank Layton, a thirty-two-year-old single male with no prior record. Hank had lived at home with his parents who spent winters vacationing in Florida. That's where they were at the time of his death. A manager at a computer games store at a local shopping mall, Hank seemed like an unlikely target, thought the detective.

In his experience, most homicides fall into one or more of three categories: money, drugs and women. What happened to Hank? Did he get tangled in a drug deal gone bad? Did he hire a hooker to share his bed while his parents were sunbathing on a beach? Maybe it turned out to be a homosexual hooker. That happened more often than people would believe.

The body was nearly drained of blood. Hank's neck had been cut so deeply that his head had nearly fallen off. It looked as though the killer had sat on top of Hank and tried to decapitate him. Chances are, it wasn't a woman, the detective surmised. But it definitely could have been a man dressed as one. It was almost always men who were capable of such aggressive violence. And if Hank hadn't known his killer, then the only reasonable explanation for such violence would be mental illness. The guy had to be nuts.

As part of the routine practice of forensics, the detective turned Hank over and examined him. But since he was drowning in blood, it was hard to find clues. Sticky and congealed, the crimson globs clung to everything. Hank rested in a body bag for a few moments before he was zipped in. The bag was loaded onto a gurney and placed in the back of the coroner's van.

While Hank lay in wait at the coroner's office, Detective Browning requested that the postmortem be postponed until his partner, Detective Chow, arrived. Then the two men donned protective suits and entered the large sterile space where further indignities would be performed on Hank.

The body was removed from the bag by technicians and placed on a shallow steel table with a drain at the foot. One tech used a shower hose to wash the bloodied corpse clean. Red water, the last traces of blood belonging to Hank, swirled down the drain.

The coroner, detectives and technicians were silent. Detective Chow was the first to speak. "Couldn't really be his calling card, could it? I know that painters sign their work, but wow. Seems kind of unlikely that he signed the murder victim, doesn't it?"

But there it was, plain as a child's new cursive handwriting. Carved into Hank's chest in neat letters were the words: *Killed by Jack Vaughn, Lower East.*

The detective peeled off his protective suit, exited the autopsy room and jabbed a phone number into his cell phone.

"Pull up the name Jack Vaughn," he said. "I'll be there in twenty."

Within seconds, they had his rap sheet. Jack Vaughn was a twenty-year-old petty criminal with a police record dating back eight years. Charges included drug possession, drug use, drug dealing and stolen automobiles. But how did this loser end up in Hank's home?

The police knocks to Vaughn's apartment door went unanswered. Noting blood on the handle, the cops were tempted to break it down but instead, they called the building superintendant who let them inside the old-fashioned way. The key turned the lock and the door creaked open.

There was Jack, sitting atop a television set. He had yanked out at least four of his teeth and was deep in concentration, working on a fifth. His clothes were as bloody as Hank's had been. Still high on PCP, he looked blankly at the officers. He had no recollection of what had transpired hours earlier.

The cops handcuffed Vaughn's wrists behind his back. Blood shed off him like dog hair. Police officers wear gloves for a reason. There was a lot going on in Jack's brain, but none of it was intelligible. As the cops prepared to escort him downstairs, he stood, his features suddenly crazed. A burly policeman dragged him to a chair and pushed him to sitting.

But even without the use of his hands, Jack, charged by PCP, possessed Herculean strength. He wound up and kicked the cop in the balls with all his might. Then, dodging everyone in the apartment, he headed for the open window and jumped, expecting to soar like an eagle in majestic flight. Instead, he plummeted to his death with a thud reserved for cartoon characters leaping over cliffs.

PCP, or phencyclidine, is more commonly known as angel dust. The dissociative drug, which makes the mind feel separate from the body, was tested as an anesthetic during the Second World War before being synthesized and sold in the 1950s by a drug company. However, because of its frightening side effects, including hallucinations, mania and delirium, the drug was pulled off the market after only a brief time. PCP has a long half-life, which means that it lives in the body for a long time. That may be one of the reasons that it became such a popular recreational drug in the 1960s and 1970s. Instead of multiple hits, a single dose lasts for many, many hours.

But as fun as those hallucinations may be for some, PCP can cause bouts of aggressive and unpredictable behavior, including the perception of invulnerability translating into attempts at superhuman acts. PCP users have tried to stop trains, cavort with lions and attack armed police officers.

Jack's family was shocked to learn the story behind his incarceration. He was trying so hard to get his life in order, his mother said, insisting that her son's actions had been totally out of character. "It was all those awful drugs!" she told the newspapers, shaking her head.

BLAST FROM THE PAST

49

Dressed in his red and black lumberjack hunter cap and flannel shirt, Rafaele scoured the forest behind his home for firewood. Then he headed northeast in the direction of an old shack that had been on the property for as long as he could remember.

Raffe, as he was known, grew up in the same house in Italy that his parents had lived in during the war. In fact, besides the few months in mid-1944 that they fled during an American offensive, the Bianchi family had occupied that house in the shadow of the Apennine Mountains for more than a hundred years. Just before the war ended, Raffe was born. When he was thirty-two, he married an eighteen-year-old girl from the village, and they moved into the Bianchi home to raise their family.

Over the years, the village had transformed from a jumble of brick dwellings full of uneducated peasant farmers into a chic getaway of summer retreats for the privileged. These days, gleaming sports cars vied for space along the two-lane cobblestone roads. It seemed that every week, a new bistro opened its doors.

Raffe lived on the outskirts of the village, far from the glitter and noise. He and his wife, Gina, had five children, but one died in infancy. They raised their kids and watched each one leave the nest. Then, just as they had become free birds themselves, Gina was diagnosed with ovarian cancer, and she lost her battle only months later. That sad day was two years back. Lonely, Raffe was delighted when his youngest son, Aldo, asked to move his own family into the Bianchi abode.

Raffe had always been an early riser. Quietly, he prepared for the day ahead, careful not to disturb his sleeping family. He tossed a log into the wood-burning stove, which was as old as the home itself and still a trusty heat source during the winter months. This house may not have air conditioning or fancy TVs but it was cozy, Raffe thought, especially for a man enjoying an early retirement.

Having toiled for years as a restaurateur, he had been smart with his money and would be looked after until he was in his grave. At sixty-two years old, he wasn't preoccupied with death. When his time came, Raffe expected to die right here, in his home, where it was warm.

This particularly bright morning, he trudged the few hundred yards into the forest, his ax slung over his shoulder. He pulled a sled behind him.

Hauling wood was hard work for a man his age, but Raffe did not even consider home delivery. Since boyhood, he had spent fall days chopping trees in preparation for the cold Italian winters. When his own kids were old enough, they had headed into the forest along with him. To start the day, Raffe would build a fire in a clearing, and while the children played around it, he would go about chopping trunks and separating branches. At noon, the family would sit by the fire and feast on the lunch that Gina had packed the night before.

Now, Aldo, busy emailing at the office, worried that his father was too old to take on the burden of such hard work alone. He had asked him to wait until next weekend when Aldo could help, but Raffe wouldn't hear of it. The temperature was expected to plummet and he wanted to make sure that the house stayed warm. Besides, he was the patriarch of the family. It was his responsibility to keep his family comfortable.

Raffe brushed aside his son's concerns, but promised to spend just half the day collecting. "Next weekend, you and I will take the little ones out and finish the job," he told his son.

For twenty minutes, Raffe marched through the brush. He was panting softly by the time he found a familiar clearing about half a mile in. He collected some kindling and then, in an untouched corner, he started a small fire. In his sack, his daughter-in-law had packed a thermos of coffee, baked eggs in tomato sauce and rice balls. The food would never rival Gina's cooking, but it was a close second and for that, Raffe loved the girl.

In no time, the fire was raging. Raffe arranged four logs

parallel to one another over the flame and sat down on a nearby log to warm his bones. Soon, he would start the real labor.

In the early evening, Aldo found the house empty. He felt a stab of regret. It really was too bad that he had missed this annual ritual. Next year, he would take off work to help his father saw and haul. He wouldn't miss the outing again.

A half hour later, Aldo found himself watching the clock. Dusk had melted into darkness and he knew that his father would have to squint to find his way back. Aldo began to pace around the house, his fear heating into anger.

"Why doesn't he have a damn cell phone?" he asked his wife. "Who doesn't carry a cell phone?"

Finally, Aldo pulled on his boots and down coat and set off in search of his father. Maybe he would meet him along the path or find him stacking trees on his sled.

After thirty minutes of searching the brush in the dark, Aldo was frantic. The sliver of moon was a poor source of light, so he scanned the fields with his flashlight, shouting for his dad. Doubling back, he followed the unmistakable scent of burning fire. Smoke curled up from the clearing as Aldo tried to ignore the puzzle of shadows the trees cast everywhere.

He did not see his father until he was nearly on top of him.

"Dad! Dad!" he shouted, bending over, shaking the man who suddenly looked so frail lying on the earth. Sobbing, Aldo feared his father may have suffered a heart attack or stroke. He called 911.

After the ambulance pulled up to the scene, the medics worked hard to extricate Raffe from the clearing in the dark. He was transported to town for a postmortem examination.

The coroner noted that the body, which appeared to be in good health, belonged to a man in his sixties. The external exam disclosed a stab wound at the level of the cervical spine. X-rays of the body showed a metallic fragment lodged in the man's brain, with the entry point at the occipital bone of the skull.

The homicide investigators were pretty sure they had a murder case on their hands. At first light the next morning, they returned to the scene of the apparent crime to look for clues. The fire was still smoldering and there were metallic fragments dotting the circumference of the campfire. Beneath the fire, there was a large crater. Blood had shot, as if from a pop gun in the hands of a child, in every direction.

The investigators were stumped. If this wasn't a simple homicide, then what? How could they explain a bomb explosion in the middle of nowhere? It was time to call in their munitions expert, Paolo Fabrizi.

Fabrizi had years of experience on the battleground. Now in his eighties, the man had spent his career fighting in the Italian army, initially in bomb disposal and later, as an instructor. Immediately upon surveying the scene, Paolo was nodding. He bent to pick a few fragments off the ground and turned them over in his palm. He knew exactly what they were.

He explained to the police that they were pieces of a Second World War–era ATM 9 antitank rifle grenade from the U.S. Army. A standard high explosive armament weighing just over a pound, it was an effective combat weapon used to fight numerous targets.

In a crazy twist of fate, Raffe had constructed a fire directly on top of the buried grenade. It had lain dormant for over sixty years — that is, until the heat of the fire set it off, blasting the metal. The fragments flew at Raffe so fast, he had no idea that as they sunk into his neck and skull, he was a marked man.

THE WOMAN WHO SWALLOWED HER CAT

50

*A cat lady was found dead in her living room. There was evi-*dence of a fierce struggle.

Early on, there were signs that something was amiss. Unopened junk mail sat in a growing mound by the front door. After a few too many days without an appearance by either the homeowner or her cat, the nosy next door neighbor had called the police.

Beatrice was a cat lady herself. In fact, she shared her home with a whole slew of little darlings. But although her cats seemed to get along fine and dandy with Jangles next door, Bea herself didn't have much use for her neighbor, Marla.

A single woman in her late thirties, Marla had kept to herself during the five years that she lived in the red brick bungalow on Strathearn Road. Bea found Marla awfully strange.

In fact, the woman was exhibiting some mighty peculiar behavior indeed.

Only two weeks ago, at three in the morning, Bea awoke to loud thumps. She had rushed outside to find Marla in Bea's very own garden. The woman was brandishing a weed whacker and had already succeeded in reducing Beatrice's days of planting to a broken heap of vegetable corpses. Even more disturbing, Marla was dressed in only her bra.

When the police arrived, for the tenth time that year, Beatrice was so horrified that she insisted on pressing charges. It was high time the woman paid for her dastardly crimes. Bea huffed as she watched her neighbor being led away in handcuffs just as the sun rose high enough to expose Marla's bare butt. When she saw Marla walk up the steps to her home a few days later, Bea was determined to become even more vigilant, to take note of the madwoman's every move.

Days later, Beatrice watched in awe as Marla brushed her lawn with giant strokes of purple paint. Each time she pulled the brush across the grass, the woman spread her arm in a great flourish.

What Beatrice didn't know was that her neighbor suffered from bipolar affective disorder, causing her moods to swing from the depths of depression to atmospheric mania. Her cycles of lows and highs had intensified over the years and recently, lost in so many episodes of mania, Marla had stopped swallowing the pills her doctor had prescribed. With no laws to force medications into her, Marla was free to wallow in the depths of severe mental illness.

Now, after putting the finishing touch on her purple

masterpiece, Marla stepped back to survey her handiwork, hands clenched on her hips. It was lively, so lively, she decided. But the backyard would have to wait. There were too many other jobs that needed doing around the house first.

That evening, Marla dragged a ladder from her garage to the porch and began to climb. It was time to get to work hanging her strings of twinkling Christmas lights. Who cared if it was mid-August! There was work to be done! People to cheer!

"That's it!" Beatrice growled to her cats, as she scrambled for the phone. "Time to commit this freak!"

But when she called police, they explained that while Marla's actions may be strange, they were not in any way against the law. It was clear that they were getting tired of Bea's phone calls.

When Marla began lugging her bedroom furniture outside, Bea knew she had to take matters into her own hands. If the police refused to take action, then it was all up to her. It was time to consider listing her house for sale. Unfortunately, though, one look at Marla or her freak show house and any prospective buyer in their right mind would run for the hills.

By the afternoon, Marla had set up her mattress and nightstands on the purple front lawn, replete with lamps and an alarm clock. Panting, Marla would not be deterred, no matter how heavy the furniture. She used all her strength to shove her dresser, its drawers brimming with bras and panties and nylons and shorts, out the door. Then, with dainty hands, she placed a small area rug beside the bed so she would have a nice and cozy treat for her feet after the morning dew.

For the next two nights, Marla slept in her new bedroom

under the stars. On the third night, Beatrice hatched a plan. Keeping watch on her neighbor's lawn, she waited patiently for the moment that Marla would sashay out the front door in her silk PJs and climb carefully into bed. Bea had her hand on the phone.

But Marla surprised her by failing to show up that night, or the night after that. At first, Bea was relieved. Maybe the woman had finally come to her senses. But after five days of no Marla, Bea's good Samaritan gene kicked in and she began to worry. The fact was, Beatrice knew the intimate details of her neighbor's comings and goings better than anyone on earth. So when Marla didn't sunbathe nude on the roof or remove the windows from her kitchen, or ride her bicycle in circles on the street, there was something terribly wrong.

Even though she knew the police were sick of hearing her voice, and even though she couldn't stand the sight of her neighbor, Bea did the right thing and picked up the phone. The police car took its sweet time meandering its way up Strathearn Road.

Careful not to disturb the bedroom, two uniformed cops made their way across the purple lawn and climbed the three stone steps to Marla's front door.

An investigator's nose is his number one tool. For these cops, there was no mistaking the scent. When they forced open the door, they found exactly what they had suspected: a corpse. They figured it was just another suicide, on another warm day, in another single story bungalow.

They didn't even need to cross the threshold. There she lay. The cat lady. Facing them in front of an old hairy couch.

The senior cop hesitated. He would be the lead investigator assigned to this case so he had better get the facts straight. Was this definitely a suicide? The corpse was covered in bloody scratches. Her face looked as if it had been whipped by a cactus-wielding intruder. Her arms and hands were scarred with cuts. There was a weed whacker lying near the body. Could the lady have killed herself using a garden tool?

The lead investigator stationed his partner at the door and began a slow examination of the scene.

The house was nasty, strewn with clothes and papers and God knew what else. Clearly, the cat lady was a classic hoarder. Stepping through the maze of junk littering the hallway, the cop entered the kitchen where again, he smelled death.

On the counter, by the sink, rested the remains of an animal. It was missing its eyes, paws, tail and so many other parts that it was barely recognizable. Tufts of gray fur were scattered across the countertop. An open bottle of A1 Steak Sauce lay on its side, its contents oozing onto the cutting board. Disgusted, the officer pulled out his cell phone and called the coroner.

After the requisite photos had been snapped from every conceivable angle, the bodies of the cat lady and what remained of her beloved pet were packaged and removed. The apartment was secured and the autopsy was planned for the following day.

The pathologist on call, Dr. Bateman, had fished out many unnatural objects from bodies in her career. She began scoping inside the woman's stomach. There, she found a cat's intestines, fat tissue and strips of fur-covered skin. Dissecting upward, the doctor discovered numerous feline parts including the cat's liver, paws and eyeballs. They were stuck in the woman's esophagus. In her throat, immediately above the epiglottis, a cat kidney had obstructed her airway.

Asphyxia is caused by either smothering or choking. In both cases, the result is the same, but the process — how the airway gets blocked — is different. Smothering occurs when there is a blockage anywhere above the epiglottis, including at the level of the nose or mouth. With choking, however, the obstruction occurs below the epiglottis.

If only Marla had paused during her manic meal, stopping before she swallowed Jangles' kidney, she might still be alive today. Instead, Marla just kept on eating, without taking a breath, thereby earning her moniker, the cat lady. Fueled by her bipolar illness, she had not simply killed her cat, but she chopped it up and then ate it raw, like feline sushi.

As evidenced by the scratches crisscrossing Marla's face and arms, Jangles was in no mood to be eaten. You had to hand it to the creature: she put up quite a fight. But the cat was no match for the cat lady who may not have thought to garnish her supper with a side of veggies, but at least had enough foresight to flavor it with her favorite steak sauce. At the end of the day, though, it was Jangles who had the last word. If she was going to die, it wouldn't be alone.

ACKNOWLEDGMENTS

Without my wife Randi's editing, re-editing, writing and rewriting, *The Woman Who Swallowed Her Cat* would not be the bestseller it has become, or rather, I hope it will become. I am proud of this book because she transformed it into a finished product. Without Jack David at ECW Press, I would never have published my first book way back in 1997, leading to this fourth book, with a goal of eventually living off literary royalties. Without my three kids Seth, Rachel and Aaron, I wouldn't need to wait for royalties.

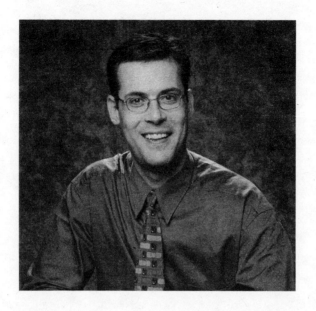

Dr. Myers is a cardiologist at Sunnybrook Health Sciences Centre in Toronto, Canada, where he lives with his wife, Randi, and his kids, Seth, Rachel and Aaron. This is his fourth book. Dr. Myers is decidedly one-dimensional with few hobbies and friends. He spends most of his time talking about comic books with Seth, picking up Rachel from gymnastics and watching Aaron play hockey. The impetus for writing this book lies in the term *gob-smacked*, as he continues to be amazed by unusual behavior and rare random medical presentations — which only serves to exacerbate his paranoia that it could happen to him.